Restoring the Temple

7 Steps to a Healthier You

Kat Ponds

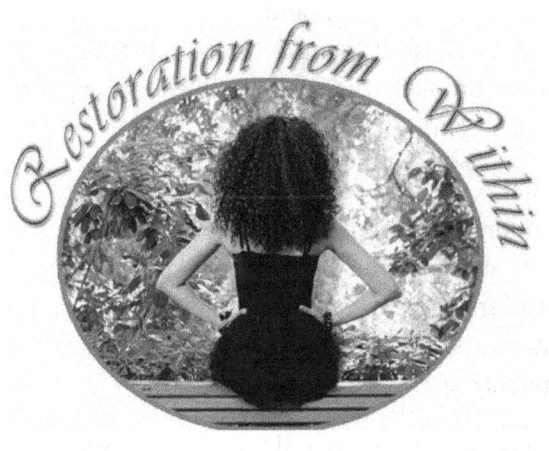

Moncks Corner, SC

Restoring the Temple: 7 Steps to a Healthier You by Kat Ponds

This book or parts thereof may not be reproduced in any form, stored in a retrieval system, or transmitted in any form by anyone--electronically, mechanically, photocopying, recording, or otherwise—without the written permission of the publisher, except as provided by United States of America copyright law.

Copyright© 2018 by Kat Ponds

All right reserved.

Limit of Liability/Disclaimer of Warranty:

Please allow the Great Godly Physician to work hand-in-hand with your earthly physician. This book is for educational purposes only. It is not intended to be a substitute for medical advice from a qualified physician. No information in this book is meant to replace medical advice from a qualified physician, diagnosis or recommendations for medical treatment of any disease. The reader should consult a physician for the diagnosis and treatment of any health-related problem. The author, publisher, manufacturer, or distributors cannot accept legal responsibility for any problem arising out of the use of experimentation with methods described herein.

Mention of specific companies, organizations, or authorities in this book does not imply their endorsement of this book, nor does it imply the publisher's endorsement of the above. While the author has made every effort to provide accurate internet addresses and resources at the time of publication, neither the publisher nor author assumes any responsibility for errors or for any changes that occur after publication.

The nutritional facts for restaurants and brand-name products mentioned in this book were made public by their companies. For companies who do not provide complete nutrition information to the public, the estimates and knowledge share about products and produce were obtained by www.cdc.gov, www.healthydiningfinder.com, www.choosemyplate.gov, www.foodmatters.com, other product websites, and "Eat This and Live" book.

Mention of specific documentaries and movies in this book does not imply their endorsement of this book, nor does it imply the publisher's endorsement of the above.

For general information on our other products and services, please visit www.RestorationfromWithin.com.

Unless otherwise stated, Scriptures are taken from the Life Application Study Bible Study HOLY BIBLE, NEW KING JAMES VERSION (NKJV), Copyright© 1988, 1989, 1990, 1991, 1993, 1996 by Tyndale House Foundation. Used by permission of Tyndale House Publishers, Inc., Carol Stream, Illinois 60188. All right reserved. Used by permission.

Also Used: Scripture taken from HOLY BIBLE, NEW LIVING TRANSLATION, Copyright© 1996, 2004, 2007, 2013, 2015, by Tyndale House Foundation. Used by permission of Tyndale House Publishers, Inc., Carol Stream, Illinois 60188. All right reserved. Used by permission.

Also Used: Scripture taken from THE MESSAGE. Copyright© 1993, 1994, 1995, 1996, 2000, 2001, 2002. Used by permission of NavPress Publishing Group.

Also Used: Scripture taken from THE HOLY BIBLE, NEW INTERNATIONAL VERSION®, NIV, Copyright© 1973, 1978, 1984, 2011 by Biblica, Inc Used by permission. All rights reserved worldwide.

Also Used: Scripture quotations are taken from the New Amplified® Bible (AMP), Copyright© 2015 by The Lockman Foundation Used by permission. www.Lockman.org

Also Used: Scripture quotations are from ESV® Bible (The Holy Bible, English Standard Version®, Copyright© 2001 by Crossway, a publishing ministry of Good News Publishers. Used by permission. All rights reserved.

Published by Restoration from Within, LLC

Ordering information: To order bulk copies, please email the author at kat@restorationfromwithin.com for bulk order rates.

Visit the author's website at www.RestorationfromWithin.com.

ISBN -13: 978-0-692-08193-8

Printed in the United States of America

Dedication

Abba,

I give you my first fruits as an author. May my light shine brightly before Your daughters, that they may see my good works (inspired by You), and they exponentially glorify Your Name. May they be inspired, encouraged, and restored from within so they can be set free to walk boldy in their purpose and destiny.

Table of Contents

Forward 9
Introduction 12

Chapter 1
God's Original Plan 19

Chapter 2
8 Temple Destroyers 25
#1 Not Knowing Yourself or The Enemy 25
#2 Lack of Commitment 33
#3 Negative Mindset 35
#4 Stress 39
#5 Not Enough Rest and Relaxation (R&R) 43
#6 No Physical Activity 50
#7 Food Additives 53
#8 Fast Foods 56

Chapter 3
The Importance of Restoring Your Temple 67
#1 Ask for Help! 73
#2 Remove or Drastically Reduce Processed Foods 75
#3 Whole Foods 79
#4 Whole Foods Supplement and More 84
#5 Increase Water Intake 88
#6 Control Sugar Intake 90
#7 There's Power in Accountability 94

Acknowledgments

Abba,

"25 Whom have I in heaven but You? And there is none upon earth that I desire besides You. 26 My flesh and my heart fail, But God is the strength of my heart and my portion forever."

Psalm 73: 25-26 (NKJV)

Dentriss, I am in awe of your steady faith as we have journeyed through this roller coaster ride called life. I love you to life. You're the real MVP in supporting me in pursuing my dreams. I will always be your ride or life Chic! #BurnRubberNotYourSoul

Tt, Ky, and Noah, as you grow older, I pray to see you fly out of the nest and into this world and soar like eagles. May you pursue all your God-given dreams. May you live life to the fullest. I know momma's tough on you; however, I love you enough to set boundaries in your life that will later be standards on which you will live. There will be times in your life when the hassles of life will get you down. Whenever your spirits become low, just remember with God as the lamp unto your feet, you will always be directed to your destined path. I will ALWAYS have your back. I loveeeeeeeee you to life! You have been so patient and understanding as I took the journey of writing this book. I pray my journey inspires you to realize with God NOTHING is impossible.

La familia es una institucion! Margaret and Juan, thank you for doing your very best to love me. I was blessed to have two sets of parents in this world. Nury (Mami) and Carlos (Papi), you made a lot of sacrifices as grandparents raising a granddaughter. It was your unconditional love, support, and old school ways that have sparked a passion for helping others, following my God-given dreams, and leaving my mark in this world. I hope and pray I am making you proud. Ulysses, no one or anything will stop my love for you. La sangre no miente, tampoco el amor de nuestro Dios que tiene para nosotros. He will never leave or forsake you, Bro. I love you to life. Charlie, Ana, Charles, and Naduah, you guys, have truly been my foundation. Words could never express my love and appreciation for each of you. Los quiero de gratis!

Bishop Jerome A. Taylor and Dr. Tonia A. Taylor: Dentriss and I will forever be grateful for how you have selflessly taught, loved, prayed, spoken life, supported, and encouraged our family. You helped us build our faith and a strong spiritual foundation on Kingdom principles. We praise God for your ministries, all of which have assisted us in realizing our God-ordained destiny. We love you to life!

To our village: Dentriss and I have prayed for each of you, and God has hand selected the BEST! You have prayed, encouraged, supported, corrected, redirected and most of all loved on each of us through the tough and great times.

To my tribe: Through each of you, I've experienced the power of sisterhood, unity, love, and accountability. I am so grateful we are doing life together. You all inspire me to live my life to the fullest. I love you.

Remnant Sisters: My life has exponentially changed since God assigned me to be part of this global assignment. I have witnessed signs, wonders, and miracles in and through each of you. I thank God for you! We are armed and stand ready for the journey God has in store for us through Remnant Warriors Global, Inc.

The BEST Coach in the World is LaVondilyn San Kitts! Don't debate me! Lol, I am so grateful for your obedience and all that you've poured into me personally and professionally. You set me on FIA, and I am genuinely appreciative.

Adelai Brown, I am super grateful that God divinely connected us to take this journey together. The healing and deliverance that took place on this journey together have been priceless.

To the rest of the 2017 Writeousness Crew, we made it!!!! Hallelujah!

Editing & Graphic Design Team: Reverend Dr. Gwendolyn Parmley-McCloud, Jasmine Hardy, and Adelai Brown. You handled the editing process with gentle gloves; crossing all of my Ts and dotting my Is. Stefany Designs I am thankful for your creative gift. Your editing and creativity has added clarity and caused this book to look great! I applaud each of you for a job well done. Thank you.

Restoration Girlfriends, thank you for trusting me with your health journey.

Forward

Do you agree that sometimes the word "healthy" can be a little intimidating?

The whole idea of getting "healthy" seems difficult, doesn't it? It requires change – changing what you eat, where you eat, how you eat, even when you eat. It even requires you to shop differently. "Healthy" seems like such a task!

I do not know about you, but the challenge for me has always been determining whether it was worth all the changes I would to go through to get to that overall "healthy" place. If that is your challenge today, let me encourage you: it is WELL worth it!

May I tell you a story?

While sitting in a local fast food restaurant not too long ago, a friend and I were having a conversation. Being very transparent, she revealed to me that she had just recently had an outbreak of Fibromyalgia – a chronic, painful condition caused by overactive nerves. As she described the pain and how it demobilized her and kept her from enjoying her life, something inside of me got so angry. I wanted to throw her chicken nuggets and soft drink, along with my chicken sandwich and sweet tea in the trash can! You see, I knew that her diet greatly exacerbated her pain. As she shared her struggle, I could only think of one truth: This is NOT what God wants for us.

I had a God-given revelation that day, and that revelation was this: Our food choices are directly tied to our ability to live or not live an abundant life. John 10:10 tells us that Christ died for us that we might live life more abundantly. But, that "life to the full" escapes us if we are always running on empty! Even though the abundant life is available to us, we cannot live it if we are depleted, sick, tired, and pain-ridden all the time. We cannot live an abundant life if our bodies are weighted down with unnecessary weight, housing all kinds of toxins, ailments, and diseases!

That day, I decided it was time to change what I consumed in my body – and challenged my friends to do the same. I decided to study and choose my food choices from a kingdom perspective striving to line those food choices up with the Word of God. The truth of the matter is, my body (and your body, if you are in Christ) houses the Holy Spirit. His spirit dwells within us! We should not defile it with sin or immoral activities. We certainly should not defile it with greasy, fat, unhealthy, toxin-laden foods either. Why? Simply, we need our bodies to function at their best, so they can perform the works God has called us to do!

My mind was made up that day to take better care of my body, choosing carefully to put only healthy foods and drinks into it! I determined that day to show God just how willing I was to live the life He died for me to live. I vowed that day to willingly line up my eating habits with my love for Him and His Word. I promised to honor this Temple, filling it with only the good of the land – good food, good thoughts, good emotions, Everything Good! I pledged to become healthy and completely restored.

May I extend that same challenge to you today? Will you begin to see your eating habits as another way to bring glory to God and honor this wonderfully made body He has given you? Will you commit to aligning your actions – even your food choices – with His Word? Will you agree to let whatever you eat, or drink bring glory to God, just as it says in 1 Cor 10:33?

If you accept this challenge, Kat Ponds is the perfect coach to assist you in fulfilling your goal. Her advice in this book is invaluable! She will help you make better step-by-step decisions in all areas dealing with your health. She will walk you through what it means to be healthy inside out. If you are ready to be restored from within, ready to begin your journey toward a healthier you, then I encourage you to grab your journal, a pen, as well as a tall, refreshing glass of water and settle in…she has so much in store for you!

Here is the truth, woman of faith: God has a great plan for your life. His plan is a good plan – a plan to prosper you, a plan to give you a hope and a future. Yet, that plan requires you to be healthy and whole. Do what you can in the natural, and He will bless your natural with His supernatural. Together, living life more abundantly will become a reality for you.

Do you agree? Good! Well, get started today.

May I pray for you?

Lord, bless this woman of faith. Strengthen her on this journey. Open her spiritual eyes and open her heart to receive the wisdom in this book. Show her just how much you love her and have in store for her. Help her to love herself enough to do only good for herself and her body. Remind her now, that you have given her a spirit of power and of love and of a sound mind. Empower her to press, "go" toward her health, never turn back! Restore her from within and help her to live more abundantly…In Jesus's Name! Amen.

LaVondilyn W. San Kitts, FIA Faith Builder™, Coach & Author

www.onFIAministries.com

Introduction

As a wife, mother, and an entrepreneur, my life gets busy and chaotic! I know what it is like to feel overwhelmed, depleted, and tired. I used to wonder, "Is this really it?" I now realize I was feeling empty and yearning for more in life. I wondered why my body ached. Why I felt like a dumping ground. Why were my body and mind always tired and frustrated?

Guess what it still gets that way sometimes. I have comfort in rejoicing in my new-found strength; I have become a seasoned warrior!

I sought God, and He has guided me into a different place. Now, I know how to combat my emotions, keeping them from being all over the place. I'm no longer confused, sick all the time with no energy. When life tries to hand me lemons, I have learned how to make some banging lemonade and sip on it with my pinky finger up!

How did I do this? By returning back to Him to His Master Plan for my life.

Are you tired of trying to figure out how to find the balancing point between it all? Are you wondering if there is such a thing as balance? Well, **Restoring the Temple: 7 Steps to a Healthier You** will take you on a tour of my journey. This two-part journey will include God's Original Plan for Your Temple and a Personal Restoration Plan for your Temple with 7 Steps to a Healthier You.

In the first part of your journey, you will discover the 8 Temple Destroyers, the importance of restoring your Temple, and the action steps needed to recognize any Temple Destroyers in your life. Next, you will step right into the second part of your journey and attain a personal restoration plan for your individual Temple. You will learn the importance of being disciplined and embracing change. We will finish this leg of the journey by learning the 7 Steps to a Healthier You. You, along with my partnering right beside you, will put these steps immediately into action so that you can gain:

- Victory
- Clarity
- Vitality
- Strength
- Restoration

Once accomplished, you will be empowered to live the life He has for you!

God desires that we have peace, health, and vitality. By finally returning back to Him, we can be redeemed, renewed, and restored.

When we stay within His plan for us – which is a good plan - then our days are better, our lives are better, and we are better!

I have put on the full armor of God [for His precepts are like the splendid armor of a heavily-armed soldier], so that I may be able to [successfully] stand up against all the schemes, strategies and deceits of the devil (Ephesians 6:11 AMP). Even before now, I have been in "warrior mode" and declared war on those strongholds that affect your life. I have been speaking against the spirits and strongholds that society and food industries have plugged into you. This "matrix" is called sick care (strategic spiritual, mental, and physical attacks on your Temple). I have been speaking to the "Temple Destroyers" in your life that is preventing you from living the life that God created for you to have and enjoy.

Would you like to know why? Because I love you and want the best for you and your family Chica (girlfriend)! I do not want you to go down the same path I had to go through to learn the importance of living an overall healthy life. In the past, I went down the opposite path God had for me and made several decisions that affected my Temple significantly:

- My body (30% chance of having children)
- Spirit (no relationship with Christ)
- Mind (low self-esteem, depression, and anxiety)
- Relationships (very guarded, isolated, and defensive)

STILL, GOD kept me through it all! Even amid my mess, He planned to prosper me and not harm me. His Word found in Jeremiah 29:11 NKJV gave me hope and a future. At last, I returned back to Him. With His cleansing power, God redeemed, renewed, and restored me! I Praise Him for being the God who gives many chances! That is what He wants for you, Chica! He wants to love on, heal, and deliver you. He wants to renew and restore all you have lost.

So are you ready to stop

- Taking pills that are only addressing a symptom and not the actual root of your problems?
- Feeling so confused that your mind is continuously running in 10,000 directions?
- Being overwhelmed and exhausted because you are unable to catch up or get some rest?
- Having your emotions all over the place?

If this sounds like you, commit right now, today to returning back to Him!

What is even more astonishing is; you are not alone in this. Many women, including myself, are walking this same journey. Many women desire to learn God's will for their overall health. These same women are serious about their family's well-being and want to transition the family unit into a healthier and greener lifestyle as well. Women, just like you, want to learn more about healthy eating (i.e., clean, natural, or organic), educate themselves and those around them about the hazards of an unhealthy lifestyle and desire healthy alternatives for their unhealthy habits. Like you, they want to be fit, have more energy and age gracefully! Woop-Woop! Can I get an Amen! Matching women of every creed, race, and color desire to be spiritually, emotionally, and physically sound to fulfill their divine purposes here on earth. You are NOT alone, Sis! We all desire to be restored from within!

It is never too late to restore from within. If you are ready to return back to God's original plan for your life, then take the first step towards restoring your Temple. It is time to join the restoration movement!

Sis, before we begin, I want to highly encourage you to make the most of this new journey you are about to embark upon. To gain the most out of this journey, you will need to become an active participant. How? By completing all the actions steps.

I highly encourage you to:

- **Invest in a health journal.** Create a quiet, secluded, and safe place to write your thoughts, challenges, and victories during your journey. Doing so will encourage you by reflecting on how far you have come and remember what God has said to you.

- **Become an active reader by personalizing your book.** Feel free to underline and highlight areas that resonate with you. Jot down any questions, thoughts, or divine insights triggered by what you are reading. You might even have the urge to respond to what you have read in the margin area.

- **Complete Action Steps.** This is where the rubber meets the road. This is where you immediately implement your knowledge and understanding of what God is saying about your Temple and health journey. For you to completely benefit from what God has in store for you in this book, you must complete the action steps. These action steps are the building blocks to restoring your Temple back to God's original plan for your life.

- **Selah Moments.** God has written personal messages just for you throughout this book. When you find these messages, I encourage you to pause and meditate on His Word. Take a few moments to ponder on what He is stirring up within your spirit. Capture these precious moments in your journal.

- **Share Your Journey.** Connect with many of the other women just like you in the #RestorationMovement Facebook group and me.

Are you ready to snatch your health back from the grip of the enemy? If so, get prepared to gain the victory over your health!

Prayer

Heavenly Father, thank you for being the author and finisher of our faith. Lord, please forgive us for our sins that we have committed willingly and unwillingly. Lord for You said that when two or more are gathered, You are present. So we thank You for being in the midst of this pivotal moment in my sister's life. I thank You for answering my prayers and divinely connecting us. I thank You for her strength & courage to want to live a healthier lifestyle. Thank You for her commitment to living in the fullness that You created her to be. I thank You that as she seeks, knocks, and asks for knowledge, understanding, and wisdom in this journey, You will provide her with answers, revelation, healing, and deliverance. I thank You for reminding her who she is in You and the spirits that You have bestowed on her of power, love, and a sound mind. I ask You for the release of her warring and ministering angels so they may minister and war on her behalf. I bind up any distractions of the enemy and his cohorts that try to come against her and her family as she feasts on the knowledge You are giving her so that she can begin her journey of Restoration from Within.

In Jesus's Name. Amen!

Chapter 1

God's Original Plan

We have strayed away. We have strayed away from God's original plan for our lives, His will for our families, and His desire for our future. His original plan for us was for good and not evil. In Jeremiah 29:11 God said, "For I know the plans I have for you. They are plans for good and not disaster, to give you a future and a hope." From the very beginning, He wanted peace and health for us. In Genesis 1: 26-28 (MSG) we read He wanted us to thrive and live long, fruitful lives! "God created human beings; he created them godlike, reflecting God's nature. He created them male and female. God blessed them: Prosper! Reproduce! Fill the Earth! Take Charge!"

In 3 John 1:2 (NLT), it states, "Dear friend, I hope all is well with you and that you are as healthy in body as you are strong in spirit." He desires for us to live a healthy life, but we've allowed life to get in the way. We have allowed the cares of this life and earthly responsibilities to take center stage. Being a wife, mom, aunt, sister, student, entrepreneur, career woman, fixer, and jack of all trades is no joke; a woman's work is never done! Helping everyone and fixing everything, always being on the move, has affected our bodies, our minds, and our spirits.

Do I have the complete answer to "fix" it? Uhhmmm, no. But I do know Who has the solution. We can find a rhythm that works specifically for us to return back to Him. My number one desire is to help you restore from within and bring you back to Him and His desires for you and your family. At Restoration from Within, my ultimate goal is to educate and equip you with the knowledge to live well, teach you to eat well, strengthen your physical self, teach you to renew your mind, manage your emotions, settle your spirit.

My Renew & Restore Philosophy will help you accomplish three objectives:

- Renew Your Spirit
- Renew Your Mind
- Restore Your Body

Most of our spirits and souls are relatively healthy and may be aligned to some degree. However, having them aligned is fruitless if your Temple fails you! How are they fruitless? Without your Temple, you are unable to fulfill your purpose and destiny (remember Jeremiah 29:11). Jim Rohn said it best, "Take care of your body. It's the only place you have to live." God has given us our Temple (body) to be good stewards over while on earth.

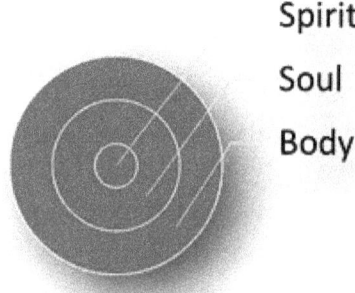

We are a Triune Being
(Spirit, Soul, Body)

As Kingdom ambassadors, it is impossible to separate spirit, soul, and body. God must take center stage in all areas of our lives. God created us to be triune/tripartite beings (spirit, soul, and body) and they each correlate with one another. When one is affected, it will manifest itself in all the other areas.

Why is it so important to you, God's chosen daughter, to live a healthier life? 1 Thessalonians 5:23 (NLT) states, "Now may the God of peace make you holy in every way and may your whole spirit and soul and body be kept blameless until our Lord Jesus Christ comes again." Hence, our body is one of the three major components comprised together in one beautiful Temple when God created us. Our body is His Temple because His Spirit resides in us. In 1 Corinthians 3:16-17 (NLV) we get our answer, "Do you not know that you are a house of God and that the Holy Spirit lives in you? [17] If any man destroys the house of God, God will destroy him. God's house is holy. You are the place where He lives."

Therefore, we are experiencing and witnessing several damaging effects to our health, such as cancer, heart dis-ease, diabetes, and many other dis-eases. Our bodies are plagued with such dis-eases because we are not taking care of our Temples. Also, we strive to have our children live better lives than we did, but many are already behind due to the harmful eating habits and lifestyle choices that we allow. LetsMove.org states, "Over the past three decades, childhood obesity rates in America have tripled, and today, nearly one in three children in America are overweight or obese. The numbers are even higher in African American and Hispanic communities, where nearly 40% of children are overweight or obese. If the underlying causes are not addressed, one-third of all children born in 2000 or later will suffer from diabetes at some point in their lives. Many others will face chronic obesity-related health problems like heart dis-ease, high blood pressure, cancer, and asthma."[1]

---

1   "Learn the Facts," Let's Move, February 9, 2010 https://letsmove.obamawhitehouse.archives.gov/learn-facts/epidemic-childhood-obesity

According to the CDC.org, in 2015 the US National Health Expenditures were $3.2 trillion.[2] The Center for Medicare and Medicaid states, "The National Health Expenditure is projected to grow at an average rate of 5.5 percent per year for 2017-26 and to reach $5.7 trillion by 2026."[3] What does this mean to you? Mo' money, mo' money **out** your pocket!

The "system" is set up for sick care, not healthcare! Guess who is in bed with the sick care system? Let me give you the tea! Many of the food and beverage companies are in bed with the sick care system. What does this mean for you and your family? Many of the foods and drinks that are consumed are highly processed and genetically grown. They are more concerned with the bottom line than with the quality of the food and beverages they provide. That's why prevention starts at home --> with you.

How can we begin prevention at home? By em***power***ing ourselves with knowledge about our bodies and how to take care of it; after that, transitioning into a healthier lifestyle (i.e., healthy eating and drinking and exercising). By taking care of our Temples, we sharply reduce these dis-eases from manifesting in any area of our triune being by resetting our Temples back to God's original plan. Oh yeah! Mo' money, mo' money ***in*** your pocket!

Ok, I can hear you say, "Sheesh Kat, we really had to go there?" Yes, because you are my sister and many of us are dying prematurely from health reasons that are preventable. Our mission here on earth is to increase the Kingdom! God has anointed you, as well as myself, to "train up" our future (Proverbs 22:6 NKJV), preach the

---

2   "Health Expenditures," Center for Disease Control and Prevention, Updated May 3, 2017, https://www.cdc.gov/nchs/fastats/health-expenditures.htm

3   *"NHE Fact Sheet,"* CMS.gov Centers for Medicare & Medicaid Services, Updated February 18, 2018, https://www.cms.gov/research-statistics-data-and-systems/statistics-trends-and-reports/nationalhealthexpenddata/nhe-fact-sheet.html

gospel to the poor; heal the brokenhearted, preach deliverance to the captives, and recovering of sight to the blind, setting at liberty them that are bruised, preaching the acceptable year of the Lord (Luke 4:18-19 KJV).

I would venture as far as to say that all dis-eases are preventable because God created the body to heal itself. Death from preventable dis-eases is becoming all too common in our current society, and heart dis-ease and diabetes are among the leaders.[4] When we decide to make healthy lifestyle choices, we sow life back into our bodies.

One of my ultimate motivational quotes is by Erma Bombeck:

"When I stand before God at the end of my life, I would hope that I would not have a single bit of talent left, and could say, 'I used everything you gave me.'"

Amen to that! I desire the same for you, Chica! Therefore, I am so elated you have taken the first step towards restoring your Temple!

Ok, so I gave you two biblical reasons on the importance of taking care of your body. Now, let us delve into some habits that destroy our Temples.

Temple Destroyers are habits that put your Temple in ruins. These 8 Temple Destroyers are not all inclusive; however, they are the ones I have seen most often. As we go through these 8 Temple Destroyers, please try NOT to place them in order of importance. They all correlate with each other.

---

[4] *"Diabetes and Heart Disease Threat to Your Prime-Time Years,"* Dr. Sears Wellness Institute, https://www.drsearswellnessinstitute.org/blog/heart-disease-diabetes-threat/

Chapter 2

8 Temple Destroyers

#1 Not Knowing Yourself or The Enemy

"If you know the enemy and know yourself, you need not fear the result of a hundred battles. If you know yourself but not the enemy, for every victory gained you will also suffer a defeat. If you know neither the enemy nor yourself, you will succumb in every battle."

Sun Tzu, The Art of War

During a worship service, I saw so many people struggling with weight management issues and dis-eases. I asked God, "Why are so many people sick in the body of Christ?" Soon after, He took me on a personal spiritual journey that will reveal several roots to the problem. Two of the root issue is that we do not honestly know ourselves and our enemy. We've allowed our personal experiences, irrational beliefs, and society to distort who we are and what God created us to be.

Knowing who you are in Christ builds a strong foundation to build your life on. It will remove the scales from your eyes, so you can clearly see yourself through God's eyes. As one of His living stones, being built up in Christ as a spiritual house (1 Peter 2:5 NKJV). You are a Temple of God. His Spirit and his life live in you (1 Corinthians 6:19 NKJV) and for you to live an optimally healthy life you must have a firm understanding of who you are naturally and spiritually.

As you take on this journey, you also return to His original plan for your life. You'll undergo a physical and spiritual detoxification. It's going to feel like your emotions are all over the place as if the chaos level went up a couple of notches, but the truth is that its part of the journey. Elimination of existing spiritual and physical toxins (Temple Destroyers) must take place so that you can remove the short and long-term effects it's had on your Temple. It's literally like peeling an onion. You'll cry, feel uncomfortable, and might not see the light at the end of the tunnel, but peeling back all those toxins in your life will help you get to the heart of the matter and allow God to cleanse and restore you from within. In Isaiah 53:5 Good News Translation (GNT) it states, "But because of our sins he was wounded, beaten because of the evil we did. We are healed by the punishment he suffered, ***made whole*** by the blows he received." God's ultimate desire is to make you whole.

As you peel back the layers, you'll uncover your true identity in God and the strategies used by the enemy to destroy your Temple.

These three areas will help you lay a strong foundation in knowing who you are and your enemy (spiritually and physically), which is researching and learning:

- Your medical history
- You blood type
- Listening to your body

Researching Your Medical History. This is a two-fold task you will need to study your family medical history (first, check out your parents, siblings, parent's siblings, and grandparents and then branch out the family tree) and then your medical history. By researching your family medical history, it allows you to see if there are any hereditary dis-eases. After that, research your medical history and compare it to your family medical history to see if there are any similarities or trends in lifestyle. Thus, you will know the "enemy" (i.e., what lifestyle did they or you have, cause, effects, and what body systems these dis-eases affect) and be fully equipped to counterattack them.

Dis-eases, food addiction, obesity, heart dis-ease, diabetes, emotional eating and other physiological and psychological issues associated with the destruction of our Temples are direct manifestations of the real enemy. These preventable dis-eases have been passed along through unhealthy habits from our culture, tradition, and lack of knowledge. Then when these dis-eases become evident, we lack the resources or willpower to implement and maintain these appropriate healthy changes. I am not saying that all dis-eases are the devil, but I am saying is that there are spiritually rooted dis-eases (Luke 13:10-11 NKJV). Please allow the Great Physician work hand-and-hand with your physician.

Once you have uncovered your family and your medical history, you'll learn more about the systems of the body and how these dis-eases affect those systems. In this new day and age, we seriously have the power at our fingertips when it comes to gaining knowledge on any subject. The internet, bible, books, and your physician are valuable resources, so use it to your advantage, Chica!

Knowing Your Blood Type. Dr. Peter J. D'Adamo's book Eat Right for Your Type is one of my foundational pillars for Restoration from Within because I firmly believe God made us unique and we should not conform to what society says who we are, but who He created us to be. Eat Right for Your Type is a comprehensive book on how the use of your blood type genetics connects the mind and body. Also, the book contains suggested food lists, lifestyle changes, exercise, stress relief, supplements and sleep patterns specific to blood types.[5] Dr. D'Adamo developed ways to further personalize nutrition and healthcare from the original book Live Right for Your Type.[6]

> Side note: Look at how God orchestrated all that through our blood! No wonder there's so much more power in His Son's blood! Hallelujah! Praise break!!!

The enemy is quite content when you are not being intentional about the health choices you make. It helps him in stealing, killing, and destroying your Temple. Thus, not reaching all of the blessings involved in operating in your full Kingdom potential.

Listen To Your Body. Your Temple is continuously communicating with you. That tension your feeling on your shoulders, headache on the right side of your face, joint pain in your knees, persistent acne in your chin area, and even the color of your urine are ways your Temple is communicating something is "off." One of my first experiences in listening to my Temple was while I was deployed in Camp Bucca, Iraq. It was a desert area and being hydrated was of the utmost importance. So, they would post urine color charts defining what each color meant in the restrooms. If your urine was amber or honey color that meant you were at high risk for heat-related injuries and needed to drink more water.

Being in tune with your Temple exponentially increases your knowledge on what's best for your health. It will also help you to pinpoint any areas that need to be nurtured or healed.

---

5 *"Live Right 4 Your Type"*, D'Adamo Personalized Nutrition, http://www.4yourtype.com/live-right-4-your-type/
6 *"Eat Right 4 Your Type"*, D'Adamo Personalized Nutrition, http://www.4yourtype.com/eat-right-for-your-type-book/

Once you discover who you are and the strategies of the enemy, you'll begin your restoration from within. It will also become easier to counterattack the other Temple Destroyers in this book or other Temple Destroyers the enemy has strategically placed in your life.

Thus saith the Lord, _____

My Hand is upon you. Because you have chosen to place me first in all areas of your life again, I will provide everything you need to restore your Temple. I heard your prayers and here's my answer. This is what you've been seeking. Now it's time for you to take action and knock on and walk through the door so that healing, deliverance, and restoration be given to you. I have created this book with you in mind. Because you are ready to learn, your teacher, the Holy Spirit, will show up. It takes faith to move your Temple from the natural (the standards of the world) to the supernatural (what I created you to be). Your faith must be coupled with action. You can no longer show me your works apart from your faith. Faith and taking action fit together hand in glove. Adjust your crown, lace up your shoes, and take action!

Things are getting ready to shift. You are going to have to change the way you live to handle what I will place in your life. You have to stop living by what "life" throws at you but live your life on purpose and being intentional. You will face some challenges, but these challenges will build your muscle. The reason why you are still here is that My Hand has always been upon you. What the enemy orchestrated to kill you, I have used it all for your good because I know your love for me. I have called you for my purpose, and NO ONE will come between you and your destiny.

Inspired by the Holy Spirit from James 2:18 MSG

 Action Steps:

Get to know who you are and what God created you to be in His Word. Start by searching for these scriptures in your Bible. Then, write them in your health journal and personalize them. Then, choose one or two scriptures per week and commit to memorizing, studying, speaking it out loud, and meditating on the chosen scriptures.

Let's do the first one together.

- Colossians 2:10 NLT

Bible Verse: *10 So you also are **complete** through your union with Christ, who is the head over every ruler and authority.*

Personalized: *I am complete in Him Who is the Head of every ruler and authority.*

Ephesians 2:5	Ephesians 2:10
Ephesians 1: 17-18	1 Corinthians 2:16
1 John 4:4	1 Corinthians 6:19
Colossians 2:7	2 Timothy 1:7

Begin researching your family's and your medical history. In your journal fold a sheet of paper in half. On the top of the right side of the paper, write "Family Medical History." List all your family's history. On the top left side of the paper, write "My Medical History." List all of your medical history.

List all of the foods your family eats during gatherings, holidays, celebrations, funerals, and passed along as tradition.

Upon completing medical lists, ask yourself the questions below and circle them with designated colors in your health journal.

Red= Negative health trends between your family and you

Orange= Positive health trends between your family and you

Black= Negative eating diet and lifestyle habits between you and your family

Green= Positive eating diet and lifestyle habits between you and your family

- What are some trends you see between your mother's, father's, and sibling's health?
- What are some trends in your family's and your health history?
- What type of diet do they have (foods and beverages they habitually ate/drank)?
- What type of diet do I have (foods and beverages I habitually eat/drink)?
- What type of lifestyle do they live (sedentary or active)?
- What type of lifestyle do I live (sedentary or active)?

Answer the questions below, in your health journal.

- What are some trends in your family's and your health history, diet, and lifestyle?
- What are some effects of these similar negative and positive trends between your family and your health?
- What are some things I can implement in my life to live a healthier lifestyle?
- How would you describe your relationship with food?
- What's your blood type?

- Once you know what's your blood type, please visit http://www.dadamo.com/.

Before you answer the questions below, please spend some time actively listening to your Temple and God.

- How would you describe your relationship with your Temple?
- What is your Temple telling you?
- What are the spiritual implications of not taking care of my Temple?

#2 Lack of Commitment

I have heard it said before that almost everything good demands a struggle. You did not graduate by sleeping your way to an "A"; no, you studied, did assignments, and attended class. You did not magically have that baby; you had to push that bad boy out with or without an epidural! By the way, if you pushed that baby out without an epidural, you are a bad mama jama. I salute you, Chica! That is what I am talking about when I say, "Anything worth having is worth fighting for." Dani Johnson said it best,

"Success demands COMMITMENT. If you are not committed, you will never SUCCEED!"[7]

Just like you committed to completing those tasks to start a business or reach your professional goals, you will need to apply the same level of commitment to your health journey. What is stopping you?

Time? Effort? Money?

Ok, so how much time, effort, and money did it take for you to get your degree? Give birth? Rise the corporate ladder? Start your business?

Maurice Chevalier asks us this great question, "What mountain are you procrastinating on climbing? If you wait for the perfect moment when all is safe and assured, it may never arrive. Mountains will not be climbed, races won, or lasting happiness achieved,"[8] if we don't commit to a healthier lifestyle.

Excuses are the nails that built the house of failure, and we are

---

[7] Dani Johnson, "One Hindrance to Life-Long Success," DaniJohnson.com, April 30, 2013, http://www.danijohnson.com/2013/one-hindrance-to-life-long-success/

[8] Maurice Chevalier, *"Maurice Chevalier Quotes,"* BrainyQuotes.com, https://www.brainyquote.com/quotes/maurice_chevalier_403796

building a Temple fit for the Holy Spirit. Sis, you have already taken the most crucial step. You left your comfort zone! Now I ask you to commit to moving forward into your health journey and do not look back.

Thus, saith the Lord, _____

> *"Forget those things which are behind you and reach forward to those things which are ahead, Daughter. By no means am I expecting you to become an expert or perfect in all this, but I desire that you keep your eye on the goal, where I AM beckoning you onward back to ME. This time you are NOT alone! All I need is your YES!*
>
> *We are off and running, and we are NOT turning back. So, let us keep focused on that goal if you who want everything I have in store for you. If you have something else in mind, something less than commitment, I will clear your blurred vision because of your mustard seed faith—you will see it yet! Now that we are back on the right track let stay on it.*
>
> *Inspired by the Holy Spirit from Philippians 3: 13-16 NKJV & MSG*

#3 Negative Mindset

In my studies, I have realized the mind is the #1 area of attack from the enemy. If we let it, your mindset can stop you from achieving the GREATNESS God has in store for your life. You must transform your thinking about living a healthier lifestyle. If you do not, it will rob you of the motivation and energy needed to accomplish your restoration from within. Having a negative mindset will entrap you. It will force you to focus on the challenges before you and rob you of the rewards of the future.

God is saying, _____

> *"Place your life before me. You have tried everything else. Give Me the opportunity to give you what you have been searching for and had yet to find. Here is what I want you to do, allow me to help you daughter and take your everyday, ordinary life—your sleeping, eating, going to work, and walking around life—and place it before Me as an offering. Embracing and trusting what I do for you is the best thing you can do for Me.*
>
> *We cannot conform to this world. Do not become so well-adjusted to your culture that you fit into it without thinking. Please, do not become so comfortable in your uncomfortable state that you do not want to move forward. Instead, fix your attention on Me. You will be changed from the inside out. Readily recognize the enemy's tactics and what I want from you, and quickly respond to both. Unlike the culture around you, always bringing you down to immaturity, I want to bring out the BEST out of you, developing you to a well-formed maturity (wisdom) in you.*
>
> *Inspired by the Holy Spirit from Romans 12: 1-2 NKJV & MSG*

For you to know what God wants and embrace what He wants is good, satisfying and created for you to succeed, you must renew your mind daily. You must make a daily, sometimes minute by minute, choice to "set your minds on things above, not on earthly things (Colossians 3:2 NIV)." Set your mind on what God says about you not what you, your girlfriends, mother, husband, or society say about you. Society is good for placing people in a box.

Who told you that you were ugly? Stupid? Fat? Skinny? Have bad hair? Too dark skin? Too light skin? Worthless? You are what you did in the past?

What constitutes this to be the ultimate truth? The truth about something is all the facts about it, rather than things that are imagined or invented[9]. According to the definition above, these irrational beliefs have been imagined or invented by you or others. You have embraced them to be your truth. Don't believe me? Get your journal, please. Let us confront these lies and finally shut them down.

---

9   "Definition of Truth," Collins, https://www.collinsdictionary.com/us/dictionary/english/truth

Action Steps

- Get your health journal.
- Fold one page in half.
- On the top of the left side of the page, write "Lies."
- Then, write all the negative thoughts you and others have imposed on you. Write down all the negative thoughts about your current health.
- On the top of the right side of the page, write "Truth."
- Then, get your Bible. Search and write down verses of what God says about you or your health.
- Once you are done, take a moment to reflect on the entire sheet.
- Pray and bind up those negative thoughts (on the left side) and lose God's Word (on the right side) over those negative words (Matthew 18:18 NKJV). Thank God for giving you the mind of Christ and seal the prayer by pleading the blood of Jesus over your mind, ears, eyes, and mouth gates.

Lies	Truth
"I am ugly."	"So, God created man in His own image; in the image of God He created him; male and female He created them." (Gen 1:27 NKJV) God looked over everything he had made; it was so good, so very good! (Gen 1:31 NKJV)
"I'll never get healthy."	"I can do all things through Christ[a] who strengthens me." (Phil 4:13 NKJV)

Sis, commit these truths to memory because the enemy is going to try to punk you with these same thoughts again. He may even try to repackage these negative thoughts and make it look different via other sources but trust me that ole slew foot always goes back to his old bag of tricks. My girlfriend Tish said it best, "We must padlock God's truth in our hearts, so we will have the Word readily available for battle when the enemy comes and tries to attack us." Your sword, the Word of God, will always defeat any enemy infiltration towards your mind. You will be able to cast down every high thought that tries to exalt itself against the knowledge of God and your identity in Him.

God is saying: _____

> *"Baby girl, this world is unprincipled. It is dog-eat-dog out there! The world does not fight fair, but we do not live or fight our battles that way—never have and never will. The tools of our trade are not for marketing or manipulation, but they are for demolishing that entire massively corrupt culture. We use our powerful God-tools for smashing warped philosophies, tearing down barriers erected against the truth of God, fitting every loose thought, emotion, and impulse into the structure of a life shaped by Christ. Our tools are ready at hand for clearing the ground of every obstruction and building lives of obedience into maturity.' AMEN!!!*
>
> *Inspired by the Holy Spirit from 2 Corinthians 10:3-6 (MSG)*

Therefore, God's truth should be at the core of our convictions. The truth does not rely on how you feel or think. It relies on the standard that is measured by the reality of something. That reality is God. We must accept God's truth internally and walk it out externally. Sis, this action step is not just an "exercise." It is a biblical principle on how to gain the victory over a negative mindset. When you allow negative thoughts to infiltrate your mind, it manifests into negative stress.

#4 Stress

Stress can be a motivator. It can be essential to survival.[10] Stress is manifested in the way you react or respond to life events (stressors). These stressors trigger physical, psychological and behavioral results. It is a part of life during good (eustress) and bad (distress) times. It cannot be eliminated, but it can be reduced or dealt with efficiently. Stress can be controlled through preparation and training.

We need to differentiate between eustress (good stress) and distress (bad stress). By learning the difference between both types of stress, we can better identify them in our lives.

Eustress (temporary)	Distress (chronic & ongoing)
Motivates you to defeat obstacles	Marital problems
Helps you concentrate & focus (i.e., for a test)	Financial problems
Helps you push harder towards a goal	Having a tough time coping w/ death in the family

From the examples above, we can categorize the causes of stress in our lives into three areas:

- Personal
- Workplace
- Environmental

Now that we have identified the difference between eustress and distress, below you will see several examples of how distress manifests itself in our Temples:

---

10   Christian Nordqvist, "Why stress happens and how to manage it?" Medical News Today, Updated November 28, 2017, https://www.medicalnewstoday.com/articles/145855.php

- Increased or decreased appetite
- Increased frustration, irritability, edginess
- Diminished sexual desire or performance
- Lack of focus and clarity of mind
- Reduced work efficiency or productivity
- Forgetfulness
- Disorganization
- Confusion[11]
- Depression
- Digestive health issues
- Anxiety
- Headaches

When we realistically reflect on the causes and effects of stress, it will provide direct insight on what is causing distress in our lives. This insight empowers you to seek out stress management techniques, such as praying, thinking positively, and speaking life!

In Isaiah 54:17 (NKJV) the Word says, "No weapon formed against you shall prosper, and every tongue which rises against you in judgment You shall condemn. This is the heritage of the servants of the Lord, and their righteousness is from Me,"

Please, circle the word formed. Now, take a closer look at the verse, Sis. The Word states that these weapons will be formed. This means you will be attacked, but they will NOT prosper! Let your enemies talk about you because guess what; they will be condemned too!

---

[11] "Stress Effects," The American Institute of Stress, January 04, 2017, https://www.stress.org/stress-effects/

Chica, count it all on joy when you meet various kinds of challenges, for all things work for the good of those who love the Lord and are called to His Purpose (James 1:2/Romans 8:28 NKJV).

Releasing Stress

What are some ways to drastically reduce and/or manage stress? Well, I am glad you asked. Below you will find some suggestions on how to do just that:

- **Set boundaries**- Quit welcoming unnecessary stressors into your life. The best advice someone gave me was "No," is a complete sentence." We will go into further details about setting boundaries later when we address another Temple Destroyer.

- **Surround yourself with a village**- Keep a social/emotional network of positive and genuine Holy Spirit filled people in your circle.

- **Me time!** Schedule time for some rest and relaxation.

Which brings us to our fourth Temple Destroyer that is a direct manifestation of **not** handling stress, which can lead to adrenal fatigue.

But first, a Word from the Lord. _____

> "Everything in the natural is paralleled in the spiritual. As you are being equipped for your health journey with your Temple, know that you need to equip yourself in the spiritual, too. Do not walk out into this world without your spiritual armor! Some of these stressors are to prepare you for your destiny, and others are the enemy's work - trying to steal, kill, and destroy you. This is a fight to the finish. I AM strong, and I want you to be strong. Take everything I have set out for you. These are well-made weapons of the best materials: Gird

your waist with truth, put on the breastplate of righteousness. Shod your feet with the preparation of the gospel of peace, and above ALL take the shield of faith with which you will be able to quench all the fiery darts of the wicked one put on the helmet of salvation. Take the sword of the Spirit, which is the Word of God. It is an indispensable weapon. A weapon created for mass destruction (WMD). Learn how to apply them. You will need them throughout your life. Prayer is essential in this ongoing war. Keep your eyes open. Stay woke and put them to use daily so you will be able to stand up to everything the devil throws your way. This is no athletic contest that you will walk away from and forget about in a couple of hours. You are not fighting against another human being that you physically can see. You are fighting against principalities, powers, the rulers of darkness in this age, and spiritual hosts of wickedness in the heavenly places. This is for keeps, a life-or-death fight to the finish against the devil and all his angels. Be prepared and always remember you are fighting from a position of victory NOT for victory.

Inspired by the Holy Spirit from Ephesians 6:10-20 NKJV & MSG

#5 Not Enough Rest and Relaxation (R&R)

I am going to be very transparent with you. This is a tough subject for me. I am still trying to embrace the great importance of rest and relaxation completely. I am a mover and shaker and find it quite challenging just to do nothing knowing there are a million and one things on my to-do list. I like to make things happen. Sometimes I ask myself, "Do I even have time for some R&R?" Trust me; I understand your thought process. However, I have also suffered significant repercussions because I have not taken the time to rest and relax. I have experienced depletion of energy, lack of clarity in my thought process, being irritable and have reacted in not-so-kind ways to those around me. I do not want this for you, Chica.

Before we discuss the lack of rest and relaxation, I want to hit the brakes and get to the root of the problem. I genuinely believe there are two main reasons why we do not indulge more in nurturing ourselves - worry and guilt. The enemy uses both tactics to stop us from focusing on what God has for us. He knows that focusing on the temporary challenges in front of us serves to wear us down. That's his aim.

About eight years ago, a RHEMA Word came to me while reading the "Our Daily Bread" devotional. God knew the difficult time I was experiencing in my life. A solution was handed to me by Paul Borden. Paul gave solid advice on how to tackle worry. He suggested starting a worry list.

Write down what you're worried about bills, your job, your children and/or grandchildren, your health, and even the future. Turn your worry list into a prayer list. Ask the Lord to work in each situation that concerns you. Pray specifically for your needs and depend entirely on Him. Yes, depending on Him. Turn your prayer list into an action list. Faith is action (James 2:17 NKJV). If you think you can do anything to remedy your cares, by all means, do it. As we turn our worries into prayer and action, Borden says, "Paralyzing anxiety can be replaced by concern for the responsibilities of life."[12]

Recently, God has given me a more profound revelation regarding worry.

He spoke into my spirit:

> *"Worry is a disguise. The truth behind the mask of worry is lack of trust. You trust me with some areas of your life but have a tight grip on others. How can I move in your life, if you do not allow Me the opportunity? Therefore, I tell you to let go and give your worries and anxieties to me. Give me everything that is making you uneasy and distracting you in life. Stop worrying about what you will eat, how the bills are going to get paid, and the kids needing new shoes. I got you! I have the cure for your anxieties. Look at the birds of the air; they neither sow [seed] nor reap [the harvest] nor gather [the crops into barns], and yet I keep feeding them. You are far more valuable than they. And who do you know by worrying has added one hour to the length of her life? You've already discovered the effects of stress, so let go and let Me take care of it, baby girl."*

Inspired by the Holy Spirit from Matthew 6: 25-34 AMP

Each day has enough trouble of its own, Chica. There is only so much you can do in one day. Please know God has your back. By letting Him know you trust Him, you activate your faith by turning your worries into prayers, casting your cares on God, and leaving them there. Also, when we seek His Kingdom and righteousness, He guarantees us that all these things (insert your needs here) shall (100% guarantee) be given unto us (Matthew 6:33 NKJV).

---

12   Anne Cetas,"*A Worry List*", Our Daily Bread, July 1, 2010, https://odb.org/2010/07/01/a-worry-list/

When we do not give God room to move in our lives, it creates a perfect environment for the enemy to set up shop and invite his cronies to join him. When we allow worry to creep into our mind, we are also inviting guilt to take residence. Guilt is the #1 trick of the enemy. He makes us feel guilty, to coerce us into thinking we are a bad wife, mother, entrepreneur, church member, minister or whomever because time is being taken for self. Do not be deceived. That is a straight up lie from the very pits of hell!

I will tell you what the General, aka my mom, asked me, "How are you going to take care of everyone else if you can't take care of yourself?" This is what I am asking you, too. You are doing a disservice to yourself and others when you do not first love yourself. You can never serve from an empty cup. Always serve from the overflow, Chica. There is a right time for everything (Ecclesiastes 3 NIV). My prayer is that He allows us to do twice as much in less time. Especially during those times, we have to grind it out, so when we rest, we can do so with a strong sense of accomplishment and peace of mind. I also pray when times become chaotic, we decide there's nothing better to do than go ahead and enjoy time and get the most we can out of life.

Now that we have uprooted these mega distractions and tossed them out of our lives let us get back to the physical importance of rest and relaxation.

An area of interest for most of us is our metabolism, which establishes how quickly we gain or lose weight. Lack of sleep can decrease the number of calories you burn, change the way you process sugar and disrupt your appetite-regulating hormones. Lack of sleep is linked to a major increase in the risk of obesity. This may partly be caused by the negative effects of sleep deprivation on metabolism. [13]

---

13   *"10 Easy Ways to Boost Your Metabolism (Backed by Science),"* Health Line, https://www.healthline.com/nutrition/10-ways-to-boost-metabolism

During the anabolic process, the R&R phase, your body regenerates and prepares itself for further daily activities. Therefore, you must complete both processes for your metabolism to be in its optimal healthy state. This enhances your ability to reach a goal to loose weight, gain weight, or just to live a healthier life.

Also, lack of R&R has been linked to:

- Depletion of energy
- Confusion
- Stress
- Heart attacks
- Strokes
- Obesity
- Depression

I know getting R&R is easier said than done and I am preaching to the choir. I get it. Remember, I am in the same shoes when it comes to the lack of R&R, but this is very important for you and all of us, myself included. This is where you empty yourself of the cares of the day, the stresses of the world, and allow God the opportunity to physically and spiritually fill you up. This spiritual renewal will equip you to:

- Fulfill your purpose and your destiny
- Take care of your family
- Walk boldly in your ministries
- Start your own business (or whatever it is that God wants to birth through you)

It must start with nurturing yourself. It must begin with taking the first step towards your health journey. Chica, this is the physical reason it is so important to rest.

I'm aware sometimes getting eight hours of sleep or even hanging out with your girlfriend(s) is just not an option right now.

Still, there are creative ways you can enjoy some 'me' time. Read on.

Set healthy boundaries. Because I am a helper and giver by nature, setting boundaries have been quite challenging for me. It has gotten so bad that my body crashed, and I was bedridden for several days. When I think about the importance of setting healthy limitations/barriers, only one book comes to mind. "Boundaries" by Dr. Henry Cloud and Dr. John Townsend, literally saved my life and has been great at helping me to set healthy boundaries in my life. I highly encourage you to read and reread this book, so that you may calibrate your focus on what truly matters in this life. Many people focus so much on being loving and unselfish that they forget their limitations. Therefore, the ability to set clear boundaries is essential to a healthy, balanced lifestyle. Boundaries are a personal property line that marks those things for which we are responsible. Boundaries define who we are and who we are not. Drs. Cloud and Townsend offer biblically-based answers and show how to set healthy boundaries with our spouses, children, friends, parents, co-workers, and even ourselves.[14]

Sharing is caring. When there is a family member(s) or friend(s) whom you trust and whom genuinely love your child/children, then you have a safe haven for their care, which allows you to have peace of mind while you enjoy some R&R.

Find a reputable mom's day out center or baby co-op. These establishments usually have drop-in-rates that are less expensive

---

14 *"Boundaries",* Boundaries, http://www.boundariesbooks.com/boundaries-books/boundaries/

than those of a daycare center. Free time allows you to hang out with your girlfriend(s), get a manicure or a pedicure, get your hair done, or squeeze in a massage knowing your little ones are well taken care of. If you are on a tight budget, get a babysitter for a couple of hours. If that is not an option, connect with or start your babysitting co-op. A co-op is when a group of parents get together and agree to take turns caring for each other's children.

If your children are in school or a daycare center, do not feel bad about taking a day or a portion of the day to do things that bring enjoyment to you. Another option would be to develop an early bedtime routine. This is what keeps the hubby and me sane. My girls are in bed between 7:30 and 8:30 every night. This allows mommy and daddy to have some individual "me" time and date nights. WOOP WOOP! Girl, we need those.

Chica, it does not matter whether you are a:

- Stay-at-home mom
- Single mom
- Entrepreneur
- Career woman

If you choose to take much needed and deserved time for yourself, it does not mean that you are selfish. Self-care is not selfish! Take time for yourself. Go out every now and then and just enjoy doing a hobby, volunteering, reading, running, walking, taking a bubble bath, hanging out with your girlfriends, or taking that much-needed nap. Whatever it is you desire to do, go out and do it! Treat yourself! Your Temple will thank you for it!

If you have a crazy schedule (like mine), tailor your R&R time to your schedule. Do it if only for 15 or 20 minutes. For instance, I am a mompreneur, so my schedule must work around the schedule of everybody in my household. A couple of times a week, I take a nap during the middle of the day. Why? Because I have to burn that midnight oil after everyone else is asleep. This allows me to do my work as an entrepreneur. Do not be boxed into the walls of a nine-to-five schedule, if that does not work for you. Do what works for you and your family. It's your time, and your schedule is designed around your tasks and needs, not what society or others may expect you to do.

Last, but surely not least, make sure you get adequate sleep. As stated prior, eight hours of sleep is often difficult for many to maintain. Still, eight hours is the suggested timeframe of sleep needed to feel fresh giving the boost needed to complete tasks during the day and into the evening hours. Remember, build your schedule to cater to what works for your family and what you desire to do.

We have covered the importance of having some R&R time and nourishing ourselves. We also suggested some ways you can add rest and relaxation to your daily schedule.

Now let us talk about another Temple Destroyer that also reveals itself negatively in our Temples, no physical activity.

#6 No Physical Activity

Your unwillingness to put forth the effort to exercise your body or have some form of physical activity will hinder you from feeling your best, having more energy, and even living a longer life.

Exercise is one of the pillars of living an optimally healthy life - emotionally, mentally, and physically. Because we live in a more technological and convenience-oriented world, we have lost the desire to exert physical energy.

Please DO NOT associate physical activity with being skinny. That is not the purpose. It aggravates me when people make this false comparison. Remember, God made a good thing when He created you, honey! Associate physical activity with maintaining your body the way God wants; not what society thinks it should be. Society has mastered the art of stereotyping. You must look a certain way, eat a certain food, drink a certain drink, wear a certain brand to be accepted or considered "normal." Really? If God wanted us to be the same way, He would have done it from the beginning. Who wants to be a copy, when God made you an original?

Ok, alright. I can imagine you're saying, "Kat, you just told me I need to get some R&R. Now, you want me to make some time for physical activity?" I know with these two Temple Destroyers, I am asking you to add more to your plate. It can be quite challenging. However, we naturally lose muscle mass as we age, which slows down your metabolism. Implementing more physical activities into your daily routine helps you to age gracefully and not drastically.[15]

According to the Department of Health and Human Services' 2008 Physical Activity Guidelines for Americans, physical activity

---

15   *"How to Boost Your Metabolism With Exercise,"* WebMD, reviewed January 23, 2017, https://www.webmd.com/fitness-exercise/guide/how-to-boost-your-metabolism

generally refers to movement that enhances health. Physical activity is any body movement that works your muscles and requires more energy than sitting or resting. Walking, running, dancing, swimming, and gardening are a few examples of physical activity.[16] Whatever it is that you can do, do it! Just keep your body moving.

Chica, all I am saying is to start where you are, use what you have and do what you can. Once you have adjusted to your current physical activity, increase it gradually to further build your Temple.

According to the Center for Disease Control and Prevention (CDC), 150 minutes of moderate-intensity aerobic activity (i.e., brisk walking) every week and muscle-strengthening activities that work all major muscle groups (legs, hips, back, abdomen, chest, shoulders, and arms) on two or more days a week, is one of the suggested time frames of physical activity needed by an adult. [17] I know 150 minutes sounds a bit crazy, but that's only two hours and 30 minutes of your week. Let's be real; we spend more time on Facebook! Ten (10) or fifteen (15) minutes of physical activity spread throughout the day is cool, too. It is all about what works best for you, as long as you're physically active with moderate or vigorous effort for at least 10 minutes at a time.[18]

> *RFW Health Tip: Consult with your physician on what would be a good physical activity that matches your ability.*

---

16   *"Physical Activity and Your Heart,"* National Heart Lung and Blood Institute, https://www.nhlbi.nih.gov/health-topics/physical-activity-and-your-heart
17   *"How much physical activity do adults need?,"* Center for Diseases Control and Prevention, updated June 4, 2015, https://www.cdc.gov/physicalactivity/basics/adults/index.htm
18   *"How much physical activity do adults need?"*, Center for Diseases Control and Prevention, updated June 4, 2015, https://www.cdc.gov/physicalactivity/basics/adults/index.htm

The health benefits outweigh the work you have to put into it, such as:

- Weight management
- Reduced risk of cardiovascular disease
- Reduced risk of Type 2 diabetes
- Reduced risk of some cancers
- Boosts mental health and mood
- Boost energy[19]

Also, dis-eases mentioned above, are becoming more common among children and teens because of the sedentary lifestyle they live.[20] When you choose to incorporate this into your health journey, you will not be the only one reaping the benefits. Trust me your kids are watching. Include them in your physical activities as well, making it a family activity.

What we ingest into our bodies also has negative repercussions to our Temple. The next two Temple Destroyers are examples of how the food we eat can/will either sow life or death into our Temples.

---

[19] *"Physical Activity and Health"*, Center for Diseases Control and Prevention, updated June 4, 2015, https://www.cdc.gov/physicalactivity/basics/pa-health/index.htm

[20] *"Health Risks of Childhood Obesity"*, UC Health - UC San Diego,

#7 Food Additives

The seventh temple destroyer is food additives.

I hear a lot of people say, "Oh, I've eaten this or that all my life. My family has eaten this for generations, why do I need to stop eating it?" or "Life is too short. I'm going to eat or drink whatever I want."

I understand the point being made; however, the quality of the food we ingest is no longer as beneficial for our bodies as it used to be. A lot of our foods come from factory farms. There is a significant difference between an old-school farm and a factory farm. Because most of what we now consume comes from factory farms, the food industry calls whatever is being produced in these factories "food." The truth is, this manufactured "food" has been introduced to so many chemicals and/or chemical additives, which makes it so critical to read the ingredients list on the labels of whatever you or your family consumes.

RFW Health Tip: The ingredients list is arranged in the order of how much of a particular ingredient is in the product you are buying, especially the first three listed. For example, if you read the ingredients list and it cites, "Water, sugar, and oil," as the first three, know that particular product has a lot of water, sugar, and oil; probably more than needs to be consumed.

Most artificial flavors are derived from petroleum. Yes, the same petroleum we put in our cars![21] Overconsumption of artificial flavors can lead to

---

21 Brian Rohrig, *"Eating with Your Eyes: The Chemistry of Food Colorings,"* American Chemical Society, October 2015, https://www.acs.org/content/acs/en/education/resources/highschool/chemmatters/past-issues/2015-2016/october-2015/food-colorings.html

- Obesity
- High blood pressure
- High cholesterol

Artificial flavors and food coloring are used by major food corporations because they are cheap, appealing to the senses (sight, smell, taste) and to give manufactured food longer shelf life. Hence, it's human-made, not God created.

Synthetic (artificial) foods are also on the list of suspicious additives. Why? Synthetic food dyes have been connected to hyperactivity, some cancers, and allergies.[22] Research suggests another area of concern, as related to artificial food coloring is that it causes a significant reduction in IQ.[23]

For example, Yellow #6 was banned in Norway and Sweden after an increase in the number of kidney and adrenal gland tumors found in laboratory animals. Yellow #6 can be found in:

- American cheese
- Macaroni and cheese
- Candy
- Carbonated beverages
- Lemonade[24]

---

22 The Journal of Pediatrics, *"Synthetic food coloring and behavior: a dose response effect in a double-blind, placebo-controlled, repeated-measures study"*, US National Library of Medicine National Institutes of Health, November 1994, https://www.ncbi.nlm.nih.gov/pubmed/7965420

23 Dr Joseph Mercola, *"Are You or Your Family Eating Toxic Food Dyes?"*, Mercola Take Control of Your Health, February 24, 2011, https://articles.mercola.com/sites/articles/archive/2011/02/24/are-you-or-your-family-eating-toxic-food-dyes.aspx

24 Dr Joseph Mercola, *"Top 10 Food Additives to Avoid"*, Food Matters, November 23, 2010, http://www.foodmatters.com/article/top-10-food-additives-to-avoid

You can see the top ten (10) food additives to avoid at www.foodmatters.com. This is one of my trusted go-to sites for continuing education. Also, if you want to have a one-on-one session and learn more about reading labels, sharply reducing your chances of bringing these harmful products into your home, I'll be more than happy to connect with you and do a grocery or farmer's market tour (virtual or in person).

Please go to www.RestorationfromWithin.com for more details on Grocery Tour™.

Artificial food coloring and flavors are harmful ingredients that can be found in highly processed foods. Many fast food industries make highly processed foods. These foods contain a lot of harmful food additives. We are paying a high price for the convenience of eating fast foods, not realizing the harm we are doing to our Temples.

#8 Fast Foods

Between building your business, career, maintaining a home and anything else that falls under the umbrella of parenting and family support responsibilities, life quickly becomes hectic. Fast food seems like the best choice for feeding the family. Dr. Don Colbert, the author of "Eat This and Live," states "Millions of people eat at popular fast-food restaurants." Although many of these restaurants have made great strides in adding healthier options to their menus in recent years, let's pause and see what is being consumed after ordering from the list of familiar favorites.

For example:

Have a Big Mac at McDonald's, and you'll rack up 540 calories and 29 grams of fat. Make it a combo and add a medium size of fries (340 calories and 16 grams of fat) along with a medium sized Sprite (210 calories and zero grams of fat).[25] Total calories are 1,090 and 90 grams of fat.

Burger King's Whopper with cheese contains 740 calories and 46 grams of fat. If made a combo plus a medium order of fries (380 calories and 17 grams of fat) and a 16-ounce Sprite (210 calories and zero grams of fat).[26] Total calories are 1,330 and 63 grams of fat.

One slice (1 serving = 1 slice = 1/8 of pizza) of Pizza Hut's large pepperoni pizza is 370 calories plus 19 grams of fat.[27] Let's say you haven't eaten all day, so you eat three slices. Total calories are 1,110 and 57 grams of fat.

---

25 "McDonald's USA Nutrition Facts for Popular Menu Items", McDonalds, July 24, 2014, http://nutrition.mcdonalds.com/usnutritionexchange/nutritionfacts.pdf

26 "BURGER KING® USA Nutritionals: Core, Regional and Limited Time Offerings", Burger King, October 2017, https://www.bk.com/pdfs/nutrition.pdf

27 "Nutrition Facts Pepperoni - Personal Pan Pizza® Slice", Pizza Hut, https://m.nutritionix.com/pizza-hut/pepperoni-personal-pan-pizza-slice/?show

According to the American Heart Association, "Nutrition and calorie information on food labels are typically based on a 2,000-calorie diet. You may need fewer or more calories depending on factors such as age, gender, and level of physical activity."[28] According to the total calories of the aforementioned fast food restaurants, we could be eating more than half of our suggested calorie daily intake in one meal. When one eats more calories, chances to gain weight increase. Gaining excess weight has been linked to many dis-eases, to include cardiovascular dis-ease.[29] Two unhealthy fats that are found in many fast foods and highly processed foods are saturated fats and trans-fat. According to MayoClinic.org, "Saturated fat raises total blood cholesterol levels and low-density lipoprotein (LDL) cholesterol levels, which can increase your risk of cardiovascular dis-ease. Saturated fats may also increase your risk of type 2 diabetes. Most trans-fats are made from oils through the food processing method called partial hydrogenation. These partially hydrogenated trans-fats can increase unhealthy LDL cholesterol and lower healthy high-density lipoprotein (HDL) cholesterol. These can increase your risk of cardiovascular dis-ease."[30]

In all honesty, most fast-food restaurants are not concerned about the quality of the foods they provide and how it's prepared. Even though the United States government is now requiring them to post calorie amounts for each food product sold, in my opinion, many are already addicted to the taste and convenience of their foods.

---

28   "The American Heart Association's Diet and Lifestyle Recommendations", American Heart Association, Updated Mar 27,2017, http://www.heart.org/HEARTORG/HealthyLiving/HealthyEating/Nutrition/The-American-Heart-Associations-Diet-and-Lifestyle-Recommendations_UCM_305855_Article.jsp#.Wnu21ainHIU

29   Mayo Clinic Staff, *"Healthy Lifestyle Nutrition and healthy eating",* Mayo Clinic, February 02, 2016, https://www.mayoclinic.org/healthy-lifestyle/nutrition-and-healthy-eating/in-depth/fat/art-20045550?pg=2

30   Mayo Clinic Staff, "Healthy Lifestyle Nutrition and healthy eating", Mayo Clinic, February 02, 2016, https://www.mayoclinic.org/healthy-lifestyle/nutrition-and-healthy-eating/in-depth/fat/art-20045550?pg=2

Fast-food providers are concerned more about their bottom line, dollar amounts. Back in 2013, a former business partner used a purchased year old McDonald's kid's Happy Meal to demonstrate the level of concern the fast food industry has regarding the quality of food its establishment creates and sells for consumption. I was truly amazed. My mouth dropped when I examined the Happy Meal. Believe it or not, the food items had not changed since she purchased it, almost a year previous. No bacteria or mold was growing on it. If bacteria and mold are not eating it, why should you or your children, Chica? My intention is not to gross you out (maybe just a little), but my heart is in educating your mind. I'm determined to educate you so you will develop a renewed mind. Once your mind is renewed, you can transition into a healthier lifestyle and become an active and informed consumer.

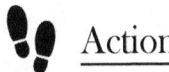 ## Action Steps

On this topic, I would prefer you visually observe the damage foods from fast-food restaurants can do to the Temple, whether it be yours or your child's.

Please take the time to watch the following enlightening documentaries on Netflix:

- Food, Inc.
- Food Matters
- Hungry for Change

Below are several questions for you to meditate on. Then journal your responses.

- What was your "Selah Moment(s)" during the documentaries? Why?
- Whom do you identify within the documentaries (if any)? Why?
- While watching each documentary, what gentle nudges did you feel the Holy Spirit giving you?
- What were your concluding thoughts at the end of each documentary?
- What are some areas that you need to improve on to restore your Temple?
- What areas of strength(s) were you able to recognize while watching each documentary that we can celebrate in your health journey?
- After watching these documentaries, what are some "take-away" you'll add to your journey to restore your Temple?

Whatever plan you choose, make it a **S.M.A.R.T.** (Specific, Measurable, Attainable, Realistic, and Timely) plan.

Write your S.M.A.R.T. plan out using Habakkuk 2:2 as a guide and reference.

Share your plan! Post your plan on our #RestorationMovement Facebook group. Your R&R Girlfriends and I are here to support you.

As we identified these Temple Destroyers, I pray God revealed to you the importance of restoring your Temple the way He intended it to be. God blessed you to prosper, reproduce, fill the earth, and take charge (Genesis 1: 26-28), Chica. How are you going to accomplish this if you don't take care of your body? Jim Rohn said it best, "Take care of your body. It's the only place you have to live."

According to John 3:1-2 (NLT), God desires that all is well with you and that you are healthy in body, as you are strong in spirit. He wants you to rebuild the ancient ruins, the Temple that has been reprogrammed to crave unhealthy foods and restore the places within devastated by:

- Processed foods
- Hormones
- Antibiotics
- The infamous genetically modified organisms (GMO)
- Food additives
- Society's definition of "healthy"

You can be free from bondage, generational curses, negative mindsets, all of which are thoughts regarding your body. Complete freedom from these bondages will allow you to know who you are in Christ- physically, mentally, and spiritually. Total deliverance from the unhealthy habits that you've developed over time because of the box that society has placed you in can now be over-powered and destroyed. Finally, allow yourself to live the life God created you to live. Move forward, with a determination like never before to fulfill your divine assignments.

As Luke 4:18 (NLT) states, "The spirit of the Lord is upon you. For the Lord has anointed you to bring the good news to the poor. He has sent you to comfort the brokenhearted and to proclaim the captives will be released, and prisoners will be free." Before you can walk into your unique, divine purpose and destiny, first you must be in alignment with His will for your life. You must be restored. You must return back to Him.

As I was researching the definition of the word restore, I found the one definition that relates best to our purpose. According to the Vine's Expository Dictionary for the Old and New Testament, restore means to 're-establish something to its original condition.' This dictionary defines the context in which we are using restore. The word originated from the Greek word APOKATHISTEMI, or an alternative, APOKATHISTANO, which is defined " of restoration to a former condition of health."[31]

Are you ready to return back to Him and experience this restoration? In these chapters, you've learned about:

- God's original plan for your Temple
- 8 Temple Destroyers (things that put your Temple in ruin)
- How taking care of your Temple is an integral part of fulfilling your divine destiny and purpose.

This is where the rubber meets the road, Chica. This is where you start treading back to Him as you develop into a healthier you. Are you ready?

---

31 F.F. Bruce, *Vines Expository Dictionary of Old and New Testament Words* (United Kingdom, Marshall, Morgan, & Scott, Publications, Ltd., 1981), 289.

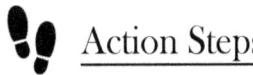 ## Action Steps

Okay, let's get it together. Here are some action steps to assist you in building a healthy foundation for your Temple. We've talked about Temple Destroyers. Now, it would be a good time to identify the root of the problem. Before you begin, let's back this train up just a little.

I would like for you to write more in your health journal. Yes, I want you to add more than just your "Selah Moments."

- In your health journal, I want you to identify your own, individual Temple Destroyers that need restoring.
- Once you identify those Temple Destroyers, I want you to write them down. But first....
- Fold the sheet of paper in half.
- On the top left side of the page, write "Temple Destroyers."
- Below it, write which Temple Destroyer(s) you need to restore.
- On the top right side of the page, write "Temple Restoration Goal(s)."
- Underneath it, write your health goal(s) for those Temple Destroyers. Also, write any revelation(s) God has given you regarding that specific Temple Restoration Goal(s) written.

Example:

Temple Destroyer(s)	Temple Restoration Goal(s)
Ex. Lack of Rest & Relaxation	• Set healthy boundaries.
Ex. God, I don't know how to say no to others/people pleasing	• Set healthy boundaries. • Understand that" no" is a complete sentence and apply it.

After you've completed your action steps above, write a letter to God expressing your desire to change. Tell God about all the health challenges you've faced. Expose Him to the good, bad, and ugly about the health challenges you've been challenged with in reference to the 8 Temple Destroyers and any others that may have been revealed to you.

Once you've written this letter, I want you to go to your quiet place and spend time alone with God. Read your letter aloud to Him. Pray to Him, seeking divine wisdom, revelation, and strength asking Him to guide you on this health journey. Ask Him to guide you every step of the way. Acknowledge that you know it won't be easy, but you trust Him to lead the way. Write down the revelation and wisdom imparted to you as you meditate and wait in His presence. Ask Him to give revelations not only at this appointed time, but continuously as you continue to read this book.

You now have the action steps for this leg of your journey. Yes!!! You are prepared to take the necessary action steps to return back to Him and His will for your life. You're ready to start laying a strong foundation needed.

I want you to please, please, please, let me know how your journey is progressing. You are not in this by yourself.

- *Email me at* kat@restorationfromwithin.com
- *Facebook:* www.facebook.com/RestorationfromWithin
- *Twitter:* https://twitter.com/KatPonds
- *Instagram:* https://www.instagram.com/restorationfromwithin/

Or better yet, you can join the #RestorationMovement Facebook group with other R&R Girlfriends just like you. It's a *closed* Facebook group where we encourage each other, share our experiences, our testimonies, and at the same time, expose each other to valuable, innovative information and insights for our health journey. Join us!

I look forward to hearing what you have to say and sharing in your journey. Don't make light of the revelations that you've received today, and throughout the reading of this book.

Write your revelations in your health journal and share with the group. We're excited to hear how you have been blessed by God's spirit speaking directly to yours!

I love you, Chica. You have taken THE MOST challenging step already.

You've stepped out of your comfort zone.

God and you have got this. Believe as you stand on His Word.

To God Be the Glory for what He is going to do through you.

Let's Go!!!!! In Jesus's Name, we move forward.

Chapter 3:

The Importance of Restoring Your Temple

Congrats you're halfway through laying a strong foundation to restore your Temple! WOOP WOOP! You are closer to your health journey goals! Let us finish laying down this strong foundation together. In this chapter, we'll discuss the importance of discipline, change, having a step-by-step plan to implement, and have a coach to help you along the process.

You **cannot** accomplish any goal without discipline. Discipline is the driving force that leads you to a target, personal success, or achievement. Hands down, this is the ultimate truth when taking on any journey in life. I am going to be very transparent with you here. Self-discipline/Self-control is another area I must fervently pray for help. There's no getting around doing so due to all the distractions that are around me. Not to mention all the daily responsibilities this mompreneur has to take care of. You know what I am talking about! My spirit is willing, but girl this flesh is weak (Matthew 26:41 NKVJ). I am already getting into the 7 steps, so let's focus on what's at hand - discipline.

The Word says in Proverbs 25:28 (ESV), "A man without self-control is like a city broken into and left without walls." A defensive wall is a fortified wall used to protect a city or settlement from potential attacks. A great example of this would be the wall of Jericho or the Great Wall of China. Self-discipline protects us from those unhealthy habits. It is a defensive wall of an out-of-control life which is open to all sorts of attacks. Without self-discipline, you're more vulnerable to attacks from dis-eases and negative stressors, thus becoming a slave to the sick care system.

Maureen Dowd said it best, "The minute you settle for less than you deserve, you get even less than you settled for." Let's not settle let's make it happen! Let's show fruit!

Once you begin to show fruit (self-discipline/self-control), you have no choice except to accept that change is inevitable. You chose to take the high road to success!

As you take the high road to success you'll gain new knowledge, a new attitude, a change in your habits (individual behavior), and influence others to join you (change group behavior) in your health journey. That's the power of embracing change. What's the big deal about embracing and understanding change? Well, it's the process you're currently undergoing. You are going through your health journey to change your lifestyle for the better. When you understand the process of change, you have a greater sense of direction.

You see, you're currently gaining the knowledge needed for a personal restoration plan. This is the easiest change to bring about. This is where you've committed to change by increasing your knowledge.

Your attitude is much more challenging to change because it has an emotional connection to either something positive or negative in your past. For example, just because you know physical exercise is critical to your well-being, that doesn't mean you necessarily agree with it. This is where discipline becomes the driving force towards your health goals.

Discipline moves you forward by changing your individual behavior. This is significantly more challenging than the last two levels of change we've identified. Old habits get in the way. It's the most time consuming, but also THE MOST rewarding. This is where the foundation has been laid, and now you begin to rebuild your Temple.

Once you are on your journey, you will see how much of an influence you will have on your family and others. You notice a change in group behavior begins to occur. Some may be supportive and join in, and some may want to stay in "This is how we've always done it" mentality. Whichever space they are in, you'll love them right where they are because your actions will definitely speak louder than your words.

Having a better understanding of the evolution of change, you have a better view to preparing yourself for what's ahead mentally. Understanding the importance of discipline and change are the beginning steps in implementing a step-by-step plan to restoring your Temple.

In Habakkuk 2:2 (NKJV) it states that we must,

"Write down the vision and make it plain…"

And we are doing just that with the personal restoration plan that was created for you. Therefore, it is so vital that you take every action step required to accomplish your health goals. By doing so, you're able to measure your success(es) realizing what areas you need to improve on. Most importantly, you're building a strong foundation. We want to be like the man Matthew 7: 24-27 (NKJV) describes; The one who builds his house on the rock, so when life's rains come, the wind blows and beats on your Temple, you will not fall because you've built your house on THE ROCK! You've returned back to HIM!

This is why God has brought us together and divinely orchestrated this connection. He wanted me to take you on a tour of my life and share what He has divinely downloaded in my spirit. God wants you to be equipped along this health journey. Chica, I am here for you every step of the way! It's no coincidence that our paths have crossed. I have been praying for you, Sis! You are one of the reasons I have gone through my journey. God has equipped me to look at your mental, emotional, physical, and spiritual needs. He placed me here, right now, for such a time as this so that you can achieve optimal health. As a coach, I will educate and empower you in self-health management and be your coach, to enable you to take a proactive approach to your health.

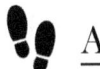 Action Steps

Fill in the blank.

- RFW Truth: Without _____ / _____ you're more vulnerable to attacks by dis-eases and negative stressors. Thus, becoming a slave to the sick care system. #showfruit

Please respond to the questions below in your journal.

> *"As you take the high road to success you'll gain new knowledge, a new attitude, a change in habits (individual behavior), and influence others to join you (change in group behavior) in your health journey. That's the power of embracing change. What's the big deal about embracing and understanding change? Well, it's the process that you're currently undergoing. You are going through your health journey to change your lifestyle for the better. When you understand the process of change, you have a greater sense of direction."*

- How has the knowledge gained in this book impacted your way of thinking?
- What changes have you made with this new knowledge?
- Do you know what path God is leading you to take?
- If you have not been able to make any changes, why do you think it's been such a challenge for you to do so?

> *"Next, is your attitude which is more challenging to change because it has an emotional connection to either something positive or negative from your past. For example, just because you know physical exercise is critical to your well-being, it doesn't mean you necessarily agree with or engage in it. This is where discipline becomes the driving force towards your health."*

- What are some positive emotional connections that are connected to your past (previous habits) with your health journey (physical, mental, or spiritual)?

- What are some negative emotional connections that are connected to your past (previous habits)?

- Has this positive or negative emotional connection affected your eating or drinking habits? If yes, how?

- What are other negative emotional connections that affect your attitude about taking the necessary steps to live a healthy lifestyle?

- Why isn't this particular strategy or other strategies working for you now?

"Some may be supportive (with your health journey) and join in, and some may want to stay in 'This is how we've always done it' mentality. Whichever space they are in, you'll love them right where they are because your actions will definitely speak louder than your words."

- What are your thoughts on not taking it personally when your loved ones are not supportive of your journey?

- How can you love others where they are at in their health journey and not let it affect the one you have embarked upon?

#1 Ask for Help!

Ok, I am just going to go right into the Word for this one. Check out what Matthew 7:7-8 (NIV) says:

"Ask, and it will be given to you; seek, and you will find; knock, and the door will be opened to you. For everyone who asks receives; the one who seeks finds; and to the one who knocks, the door will be opened."

There's great power in prayer. Look at how God answered my prayer for you. He is faithful!

In Isaiah 41:10 (NIV) it states, "So do not fear, for I am with you; do not be dismayed, for I am your God. I will strengthen you and help you; I will uphold you with my righteous right hand."

Ask for His strength and courage for the journey.

Seek Him for power and self-control. Second Timothy 1:7 (NIV) says, "For the Spirit God gave us does not make us timid, but gives us power, love, and self-discipline."

Keep "knocking" at His door for wisdom. He's eager to open the door. In Jeremiah 33:3 (NKJV) He says, "Call to Me, and I will answer you, and show you great and mighty things, which you do not know."

These scriptures are proof that God is ready and willing to support you in every way possible.

God is saying: _____

> *"...The words that come out of my mouth will not come back empty-handed.*
>
> *They'll do the work I sent them to do; they'll complete the assignment I gave them. Quit trying to do this by yourself. I*

mean how has that worked out for you? I put the possible in impossible. With Me, you can do anything. You are not just asking anyone; you're asking THE ONE who 'supplies all your needs according to His riches and glory through Christ Jesus!'"

Inspired by the Holy Spirit from Isaiah 55:11 (MSG) & Philippians 4:19 (NKJV)

If we go back to Matthew 7 (NIV) and go a little further down, verse 11 says, "If you, then, though you are evil, know how to give good gifts to your children, how much more will your Father in heaven give good gifts to those who ask him!"

Get yourself out the way and just ask, Chica.

#2 Remove or Drastically Reduce Processed Foods

Processed foods were introduced sometime in the 1940's. M&M's was one of the first processed "food" created around this time. FoodProcessing.com states, "M&M's Plain Chocolate Candies were first introduced during these times. Legend has it they were developed so soldiers could eat candy without getting their hands sticky."[32]

Processed foods are packaged in boxes, cans or bags. These foods need to be processed extensively to be edible and are not found as is in nature. Food goes through many complicated processing steps. Processed foods often contain additives, artificial flavorings, and other chemical ingredients.[33] These additives were addressed in our Temple Destroyer list.

How to recognize processed foods:

You can determine if food has been processed by the ingredients list. The rule of thumb when grocery shopping is if it has more than five (5) ingredients, and the words found in the label sound like someone is speaking in tongues; the item is processed. Honey, those tongues are not of God. Ha!

Another area of concern is refined foods. Refined grains have been milled, a process that removes the bran and germ. This is done to give grains a finer texture and improve their shelf life, but it also removes dietary fiber, iron, and many B vitamins.[34]

---

32   Diane Toops, *"Food Processing: A History",* Food Processing, October 5, 2010, https://www.foodprocessing.com/articles/2010/anniversary/

33   Fred Decker, *"Processed Food Definition", http://healthyeating.sfgate.com/processed-food-definition-2074.html*

34   *"My Plate: Food Groups",* United States Department of Agriculture, 2012, https://healthymeals.fns.usda.gov/hsmrs/EY/nutphysi/nutphysi/tn_03_02_0020.htm

Some examples of refined grain products are:

- White flour
- White bread
- White rice

What this means is many of the vital nutrients that our bodies need have been removed through the refining process. Also, refined foods are bleached and enriched. Bleached is self-explanatory, but enriched means certain B vitamins (thiamin, riboflavin, niacin, and folic acid) and iron are added back after processing the food. Since they've taken away God's natural nutrients, they have to find another human-made process, to add human-made nutrients.

Applying this information to your life will help you eliminate or drastically reduce these processed or refined foods that your family is ingesting. The Restoration Coach is here to help.

One helpful way to eliminate these harmful toxins is to go on a Grocery Tour. You and I can go on a grocery tour together. I will help you do a pantry assessment, teach you how to read labels, and develop a plan to transition to a healthier lifestyle. Go to the RFW Marketplace on my website and check out all that the grocery tour has to offer. Here are a few of the benefits of going on a grocery tour:

- Introduce more whole foods to your diet.
- Have the option of choosing a healthier alternative such as an organic or natural product.
- Save money while shopping for healthy foods.

Action Steps:

Go to your food pantry and choose five (5) foods with a nutrition label.

Once you have chosen five (5) items from your pantry, go back to Temple Destroyer #7: Food Additives. See if you recognize any of the food additives mentioned in the Temple Destroyer #7.

In your health journal, fold a new page into three sections.

On the top left, write "Food." In this section, you'll write the name of the food whose ingredient list you are to inspect.

On the top middle section, write "Food Additive." In this section, you'll write the food additives found in your food item.

On the top right-hand section, you'll write a "Healthy Alternative." In this section, you'll research a healthy alternative to the chosen processed food that you are currently eating or drinking. Write the ingredients in the parenthesis of a healthy alternative selected.

Ex.

Food	Food Additives	Healthy Alternative
Regular Brand Mostaccioli[35]	Enriched durum semolina, niacin, ferrous sulfate (iron), thiamine mononitrate, riboflavin, folic acid	100 % Wheat Brand (Whole Durum Wheat Flour)[36]

---

35   "*Publix Mostaccioli Rigate*", Publix, http://www.publix.com/pd/publix-mostaccioli-rigate/RIO-PCI-100621

36   "*Publix Penne, 100% Whole Grain*", Publix, http://www.publix.com/pd/publix-penne-100-whole-grain/RIO-PCI-137555

Now you have five (5) healthy alternatives to add to your health journey.

Once you've made these five (5) food items part of your staple, choose (5) more food items and repeat.

Our next step will help you immensely in choosing healthy alternatives.

 # 3 Whole Foods

Whole foods are foods that are unprocessed and unrefined, or minimally processed and refined before being consumed. Examples of whole foods are fruits, veggies, legumes, nuts, seeds, and whole grains (that have not been refined).

WebMD.com states, "Many studies have found that a diet high in healthy foods like fruits, vegetables, and whole grains are associated with a reduced risk of dis-eases such as:

- Cardiovascular disease
- Many types of cancers
- Type 2 diabetes[37]

God specially created whole foods for our Temples. Our bodies know exactly what to do when we eat these foods, such as heal, restore, or energize.

God didn't place Adam & Eve in McDonald's, Arby's, or at a Monsanto laboratory. He placed them on the land in which "Yahweh God planted a garden," whereupon His creation "He put the man whom He had formed" (Genesis 2:8 NKJV). God created foods such as fruits, vegetables, nuts, and whole grains to be our true source of medicine. If you've noticed, many great healthy diets are plant-based. Why? Fruits detoxify the body and veggies heal it. Our bodies don't know what to do with all these "magic pill" diets, medicines, or human-made vitamins, but it instantly goes to work when we feed it whole foods.

The benefits of eating more fruits and veggies are:

- Healthier, faster-growing hair & nails

---

37   "Phytonutrients", Web MD, October 28, 2016, https://www.webmd.com/diet/guide/phytonutrients-faq#1

- Healthier, beautiful glowing skin
- Increased energy

The best way to enjoy the healthiest form of whole foods is to buy local organic, natural, or grow your own. If you buy local, you'll know your farmer and how they go about growing their produce. On the other hand, you can have full access to your produce and control what goes into the growing process when you grow your own.

When you choose to incorporate more whole foods into your lifestyle, you are choosing to eat clean and increase your optimal health. Choosing to eat clean means to eat more whole foods because they are God created foods (closer to nature) rather than highly processed food (human-made foods).

From here people choose the path that fits with their beliefs about clean eating and their new lifestyles, such as organic, vegetarian and its many variations, 80/20 rule, or others. Below I will define the ones mentioned above, so you're familiar with these terms as you may choose to incorporate them into your new lifestyle.

Organic:

According to the USDA, organic food is produced by farmers who emphasize the use of renewable resources and the conservation of soil and water to enhance environmental quality for future generations. Organic meat, poultry, eggs, and dairy products come from animals that are given no antibiotics or growth hormones.[38]

Vegetarian:

A person who does not eat meat and any other animal product, especially for moral, religious, or health reasons.[39] Some vegetarians also exclude dairy, some don't, and some may consume eggs.

---

38   Mary V. Gold, *"Organic Production/Organic Food: Information Access Tools",* United States Department of Agriculture, June 2007, https://www.nal.usda.gov/afsic/organic-productionorganic-food-information-access-tools

39   *"Vegetarian",* English Oxford Living Dictionaries, https://en.oxforddictionaries.com/definition/vegetarian

Vegan:

Vegan is similar to the vegetarian diet that excludes meat, eggs, dairy products and all other animal-derived ingredients.[40]

Raw Vegan/Raw Food

A raw vegan diet consists of unprocessed vegan foods that have not been heated above 115 degrees Fahrenheit (46 degrees Celsius). "Raw foodists" believe that foods cooked above this temperature have lost a significant amount of their nutritional value and are harmful to the body.[41]

Alkaline Diet:

An alkaline diet consists of high alkaline foods such as fresh vegetables, fruits and unprocessed plant-based sources of proteins for example — result in a more alkaline urine pH level, which helps protect healthy cells and balance essential mineral levels.[42] Most fruits and vegetables, soybeans and tofu, and some nuts, seeds, and legumes are alkaline-promoting foods, so they're fair game.

Dairy, eggs, meat, most grains, and processed foods, like canned and packaged snacks and convenience foods are (highly processed foods). They fall on the acidic side and are not allowed. Most alkaline diet sources also state you shouldn't drink alcohol or caffeine, either.[43]

---

40   Dr. Edward Group DC, NP, DACBN, DCBCN, DABFM , *"Vegan vs. Vegetarian: Differences and Similarities",* Global Healing Center Live Healthy, Updated December 4, 2015, https://www.globalhealingcenter.com/natural-health/vegan-vs-vegetarian/?gclid=CjwKCAiAjuPRBRBxEiwAeQ2QPmwH3w04m6W-cuvElcrgVwOPNR8dvSWg9P6z2m5YqkyXwJezE888RxoCQjQQAvD_BwE

41   Jolinda Hackett, *"Types of Vegetarians",* the spruce, Updated September 21, 2017, https://www.thespruce.com/types-of-vegetarians-3378611

42   *"Alkaline Diet: The Key to Longevity and Fighting Chronic Disease?",* Dr Axe Food is Medicine, https://draxe.com/alkaline-diet/

43   Sonya Collins, *"Alkaline Diets",* Web MD, https://www.webmd.com/diet/a-z/alkaline-diets

Sebian Diet:

Dr. Sebi developed his African Bio-Mineral Balance herbal compounds and nutritional guide to support the healthy expression of the African genome. The Sebian diet is centered on the consumption of natural alkaline plant foods. The herbal compounds working in conjunction with Dr. Sebi's nutritional guideline have been known to give the body the proper environment to achieve optimal health. [44]

80/20 Principle:

My family and I began our health journey with the 80/20 Principle. This principle means we eat nutrient-dense foods 80% of the time. Eat what you want the remaining 20% of the time as you transition into establishing healthier eating habits. Once you've established mindful eating habits, you increase your nutrient-dense food intake and decrease the foods you want to eat until you are eating healthy 100% of the time.

---

[44] Aqiyl Aniys, *"Dr. Sebi's African Bio Mineral Balance",* Alkaline Based Plant Diet, Modified June 23, 2017, http://www.naturallifeenergy.com/dr-sebi-african-bio-mineral-balance/

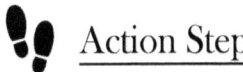 Action Step

Please watch a documentary on Netflix:

- Soul Food Junkies

Below are several questions for you to meditate on and journal your responses.

- What was your "Selah Moment(s)" during the documentaries? Why?

- Whom do you identify with in the documentary (if any)? Why?

- While watching the documentary, what gentle nudges did you feel the Holy Spirit giving you?

- What were your concluding thoughts at the end of the documentary?

- What are some areas that you need to improve on to restore your Temple?

- What areas of strength(s) were you able to recognize while watching the documentary that we can celebrate in your health journey?

- After watching the documentary, what are some "take-away" you'll add to your journey to restore your Temple

Whatever plan you choose, make it a **S.M.A.R.T.** (Specific, Measurable, Attainable, Realistic, and Timely) plan.

Write your S.M.A.R.T. plan out (Habakkuk 2:2).

Share your plan! Post your plan on our #RestorationMovement Facebook group. Your R&R Girlfriends and I are here to support you. Sharing your plan encourages us too, Chica.

#4 Whole Foods Supplement and More

Whole food supplements are derived from natural sources such as plants, fruits, and vegetables. They are not synthetically made like regular supplements. Synthetic is defined as noting or about compounds formed through a chemical process by human agency, as opposed to those of natural origin: synthetic vitamins; synthetic fiber.[45]

For example, an isolated, synthetic vitamin is made to try to copycat the vitamin's benefits found in whole foods. However, a single whole food vitamin is derived from God created sources that provide micronutrients, macronutrients, phytonutrients, and enzymes to create a synergy for optimal health.[46] This also applies to using botanical herbs as supplements, too.

Herbal medicine is known for its healthy properties which use plant or plant-derived medicine preparations to treat, prevent, or reverse various health conditions and ailments. For example, sea moss is considered a super nutritious herb because it contains approximately 90 of the 102 minerals that your body is made of. Another super nutritious herb is nettles because it contains vitamins A, C, D, K, potassium, calcium, and iron.[47]

This does not mean that supplements take the place of eating whole foods. You ultimately get all your vitamins and minerals from eating whole foods. So why do you even need whole food supplements? Factors such as:

---

[45] "*Synthetic*", Dictoriany.com, http://www.dictionary.com/browse/synthetic

[46] "*Whole Food Vitamins vs Synthetic Vitamins – What's the difference?*", Nature's Way, http://www.naturesway.com.au/article/whole-food-vitamins-vs-synthetic-vitamins-whats-difference/

[47] Aremisa May-Hailey, I.R.I.E Women's Herbal Intensive Module 3 (Dallas, IRIE Herbal Education), 9

- Food is highly processed and refined
- Reduction of nutrients from some cooking methods
- Being depleted of nutrients due to overuse of soil
- Lifestyle choices

Are all reasons why the need to incorporate whole food supplements, herbs, and other health supplements for optimal health. Think of these types of supplements as gap insurance for your Temple.

I have created a chart with some whole food supplements that will help with your health journey. Being certified in women's herbal intensive, I have also added some herbs to increase your optimal health, too.

* This is NOT an all-inclusive list of whole food supplements or herbs. However, I am sharing my personal experience and extensive research on the benefits that these products provide for our Temple. *I am NOT a doctor; therefore, I do not diagnose illnesses or prescribe pharmaceuticals. *

Whole Food Supplement	Benefits
Garden of Life: Raw Organic Meal[48]	Organic shake & meal replacement
	Raw whole food protein, fiber blend, probiotic, enzymes blend.
	It's vegan, gluten free, dairy free, soy free, non-GMO.
Nature's Plus: Hema Plex[49]	Activated with 85 mg amino acid chelated iron per serving of 3 soft gels, 300 mg vitamin C, essential cofactors.
	Hema Plex is the ultimate total blood support formula superior antioxidant protection.
	Helps with anemia and it's a vegan product.
Probiotics[50]	Restores beneficial bacteria to the digestive tract for good gut health.
	Approximately 80% of our immune system in your digestive system
	Best sources are multiple strands to include Lactobacillus & Bifidobacterium strands in probiotics.
	* Look for a potency count (CFUs or "colony forming units") of 50 billion or higher. That's how many bacteria you will receive per dose.

---

48   *"Health Meal On-The-Go",* Garden of Life, https://www.gardenoflife.com/content/product/why-choose-raw-organic-meal/?gclid=EAIaIQobChMIyOT1r-WX2QIVQiSBCh3wgACXEAAYAiAAEgJf8fD_BwE

49   *"Hema-Plex® Vcaps®"*, Natures Plus, https://naturesplus.com/products/productdetail.php?productNumber=3772

50   *"A Guide to Probiotics-7 Facts You Should Know",* Dr. Mercola Premium Products, http://probiotics.mercola.com/probiotics-facts.html

Maca powder (herb)	Balances hormones
	Increases libido
	Vitamins/Minerals
Black Cohosh (herb)	Helps with menopause
	Considered a hormone replacement (hysterectomy)
	Anti-Inflammatory
	Antispasmodic (cramps)
	Powerful painkiller
Cinnamon (spice)	Antibacterial
	Antioxidant
	Promotes heart health
	Fights diabetes
Fenugreek (herb/spice)[51]	Digestive Aid
	Lowers blood pressure
	Natural expectorant
	Increases milk production for breastfeeding

---

[51] Aremisa May-Hailey, I.R.I.E Women's Herbal Intensive Module 3 (Dallas, IRIE Herbal Education), 9

#5 Increase Water Intake

According to MayoClinic.com, "Nearly all of the major systems in your body depend on water," and it makes up approximately 70-80% of our Temple. Also, water is integral to detoxifying our bodies. Water is one of the oldest forms of detoxing your Temple. It stimulates your liver, kidneys, and digestive organs, which are known as your primary detox organs. Hence, the importance of drinking water.

Some of the benefits of drinking water are:

- Stronger immunity (detox)
- Glowing complexion
- Clear skin
- Weight loss

Hello! I am down with that! As a matter of fact, where's my water?

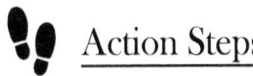 ## Action Steps

Calculate how much water you should be drinking every day.

Suggested daily intake is half your body weight.

First, you divide your body weight by two.

Second, divide the total by 8 (ounces per cup), and that's how many cups you should be drinking per day.

Be sure to add some lemon juice to your water to increase your alkalinity. Lemon juice is considered a high alkaline food, which helps the body to maintain an optimal healthy state.

Ex. 160 lbs. ÷ 2 = 80 ÷ 8 oz. = 10 cups per day

#6 Control Sugar Intake

About four years ago, my husband and I began doing the Daniel Fast at the start of every year. One of the items you eliminate during the fast is added sugar. This was the most challenging part of the fast because most foods and beverages have a lot of sugar in them. The fact that the many foods and drinks have so much sugar peaked my curiosity, so I began doing some research.

Dr. Mercola states that based on USDA estimates, the average American consumes 12 teaspoons of sugar a day, which equates to about **two tons** of sugar during a lifetime. Why we eat this much sugar is not difficult to understand- it tastes good and gives us pleasure by triggering an innate process in the brain via dopamine and opioid signals.

Therefore, you get an extreme rush when you consume soda, candy, energy drinks, and then crash after ingesting. He goes on to state, "If you are not able to immediately use the sugar by engaging in intense physical activity then one of the ways your body avoids dangerously elevated blood sugar levels is through converting those excess carbohydrates into excess body fat. This fat builds up primarily in your belly."[52]

Not all sugar is bad for you. We have natural sugars, such as fruits and whole wheat grain. However, we still need to be mindful of how much we are daily eating. Below you'll find other sweet alternatives:

- Organic coconut palm sugar
- Organic stevia
- Raw honey

---

52   *"Six Surprising Foods with More Sugar than a Twinkie",* Mercola Take Control of Your Health, May 02, 2012, https://articles.mercola.com/sites/articles/archive/2012/05/02/sugar-leads-to-obesity.aspx

- Dates
- Organic unrefined honey

Dr. Mark Hyman further explains the dangers of artificial sweeteners, "High fructose corn syrup is almost always a marker of poor-quality, nutrient-poor, disease-creating industrial food products or 'food-like substances.'"[53] Which we can translate to highly processed food.

Here are some other hazards to sugar:

- Artificial sweeteners, gum, and diet sodas have aspartame which turns into formaldehyde once ingested into your body. Yes, we are talking about the same thing that they put inside dead bodies for embalming.[54]
- Increases chances of cardiovascular dis-eases[55]
- The main cause of obesity and Type II diabetes[56]
- Overworking your kidneys while they are trying to balance your glucose levels

Also, sugar makes your body more acidic. This means it creates a breeding ground for sickness and dis-eases.

---

53   Mark Hyman, MD, *"5 Reasons High Fructose Corn Syrup Will Kill You"*, http://drhyman.com/blog/2011/05/13/5-reasons-high-fructose-corn-syrup-will-kill-you/

54   *"Artificial Sweeteners -- More Dangerous Than You Ever Imagined,"* Mercola Take Control of Your Health, October 13, 2009, https://articles.mercola.com/sites/articles/archive/2009/10/13/artificial-sweeteners-more-dangerous-than-you-ever-imagined.aspx

55   "The sweet danger of sugar," Harvard Health Publishing Harvard Medical School, May 2017, https://www.health.harvard.edu/heart-health/the-sweet-danger-of-sugar

56   "Type 2 diabetes," Mayo Clinic, https://www.mayoclinic.org/diseases-conditions/type-2-diabetes/symptoms-causes/syc-20351193

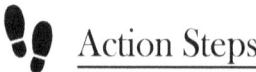 Action Steps

Watch the documentary below on Netflix:

- Fed Up

Soon after, write your response to the questions below in your health journal.

- What was your "Selah Moment(s)" during the documentaries? Why?
- Whom do you identify with in the documentary (if any)? Why?[57]
- While watching the documentary, what gentle nudges did you feel the Holy Spirit giving you?
- What were your concluding thoughts at the end of the documentary?
- What are some areas that you need to improve on to restore your Temple?
- What areas of strength(s) were you able to recognize while watching the documentary that we can celebrate in your health journey?
- After watching the documentary, what are some "take-away" you'll add to your journey to restore your Temple?

Whatever plan you choose, make it a **S.M.A.R.T.** (Specific, Measurable, Attainable, Realistic, and Timely) plan.

Write your S.M.A.R.T. plan out (Habakkuk 2:2).

---

57 "17 Questions To Ask When Watching A Documentary." *Lausanne Media Network Engagement.* N.p., n.d. Web. 12 Mar. 2018 <http://engagingmedia.info/17-questions-ask-watching-documentary/>.

Share your plan! Post your plan on our #RestorationMovement Facebook group. Your R&R Girlfriends and I are here to support you, Chica.

#7 There's Power in Accountability

In Ecclesiastes 4:9-12 (NIV) it states, "Two are better than one because they have a good reward for their labor: If either of them falls, one can help the other up. But pity anyone who falls and has no one to help them up. Also, if two lies down together, they will keep warm. But how can one keep warm alone? Though one may be overpowered, two can defend themselves. A cord of three strands is not quickly broken." It is evident in Genesis 2:18 (NKJV) that we are relational beings. We were never created to be alone.

The Word says in Proverbs 27:17 (NKJV), "As iron sharpens iron, so one person sharpens another." When you rub two iron blades together, the edges become sharper. This helps in making them both efficient at cutting.[58] If we can see the mutual benefit sharpening provides for an object, just imagine what it can do for you and your accountability partner (AP). Your AP can be your hubby, a co-worker, or a girlfriend.

On average it takes 21 days to develop a habit. There's nothing like having someone encouraging, loving, motivating, and giving you some tough love along the way. Also, you'll have your R&R Girlfriends in our Facebook group for support, too. Check out what some of our R&R Girlfriends are saying about having an AP:

> *"It makes a great deal of impact. For me, having an AP serves as a reminder to keep on track as well as a friend to go through the process with me. I am better equipped for success when someone is holding me accountable and pushing me to deliver my best."*[59]
>
> *Donloyn*

---

58   "What does it mean that iron sharpens iron?", gotQuestions?org, https://www.gotquestions.org/iron-sharpens-iron.html

59   Donloyn Leduff Gadson, "QOTD: How much of an impact does having an accountability partner make towards accomplishing your health goals?," #RestorationMovement, https://www.facebook.com/photo.php?fbid=10155856921534025&set=g.152956238246399&type=1&theater&ifg=1

"I have found having an AP has been very beneficial. It helps me to stay focused on my goals. And it also feels good to help encourage them to meet their goals also. So, it is a win situation."[60]

April

"When we sharpen one another in real Christian fellowship, the Lord bends an ear from heaven and is pleased. Not one word about Him which brings Him glory escapes His notice."[61] There is a guaranteed blessing when two or more gather in the Lord's name because He is among them (Matthew 18:20 NKJV).

Remember a cord of three strands (you, your AP, and God) is NOT quickly or easily broken. Imagine when a group of women come together; it is a restoration movement!

---

60 April Beetkah Jacobs, "QOTD: How much of an impact does having an accountability partner make towards accomplishing your health goals?," #RestorationMovement, https://www.facebook.com/photo.php?fbid=10155856921534025&set=g.152956238246399&type=1&theater&ifg=1

61 "What does it mean that iron sharpens iron?", gotQuestions?org, https://www.gotquestions.org/iron-sharpens-iron.html

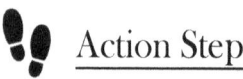 Action Steps

"The Word says in Proverbs 27:17 (NKJV), 'As iron sharpens iron, so one person sharpens another.' When you rub two iron blades together the edges become sharper. This helps in making them both efficient at cutting. If we can see the mutual benefit sharpening provides for an object, just imagine what it can do for you and your accountability partner (AP)."

- Pray and ask God to hand select your accountability partner.

Here are some suggested qualities to look for in an AP:

- Someone who has time to invest in your goals.
- Someone who is interested in growth.
- Someone you can be open and sincere with to express your strengths and areas needing improvement.
- Someone who has the courage to tell you the truth in love.
- Someone who will pray, fast, exercise, and eat healthy with you.

There's great power in the connection of an accountability partner. It helps you reach the finish line.

Finish Line Ahead

A lot was covered in these chapters.

First, we discussed the importance of discipline and change.

Second, we talked about how success is determined by taking the necessary steps to restore your Temple. Focusing on anything other than restoring your Temple is setting yourself up for failure.

Third, we rolled right into the 7-step plan to a healthier you.

Here is a quick recap of those steps:

- Just Ask!
- Remove or Drastically Reduce Processed Foods
- Add Whole Foods
- Supplement Whole Food
- Hydrate!
- Control Sugar Intake
- Power of Accountability

Are you ready to implement these 7 steps to a healthier you?

Are you ready to live the life that God intended for you to live?

This life is filled with hope, prosperity, and a healthy future. You can expect to live an abundant life filled with:

- Vitality
- Energy
- Clarity

- Sound mind
- Spirit

Become who God created you to be and fulfill your purpose and destiny so your light can brightly shine before men and women, that they may see your good works and glorify your Father which is in heaven (Matthew 5:16 NKJV/emphasis mine).

I want you to look forward to aging gracefully, not drastically, seeing your grandkids and enjoying your prime-time years. Think about what Erma Bombeck said, "When I stand before God at the end of my life, I want not to have a single bit of talent left, and I could say, 'I used everything you gave me Lord.'"

Hey Chica,

Thank you so much for allowing me the opportunity to take this journey with you. I look forward to reading, chatting, and continuing to share what God has laid upon my heart for your health journey. If you've enjoyed this book, please drop by the Amazon listing and leave a review. I really look forward to reading about your experience.

I challenge you to implement these steps into your life, and I would love it if you would allow me to continue this journey with you. To stay connected with me, you can join other R&R Girlfriends and me on our #RestorationMovement Facebook group.

Once you have laid the foundation for restoring your Temple, we can take a step further and go on a grocery or farmer's market tour where I will guide you in areas such as:

- Food assessment
- Pantry assessment
- Health goals
- Basic meal planning
- Learn how to interpret labels

To learn more about the Grocery Tour™ and other products and services, please visit my **RFW Marketplace** at ***www.RestorationfromWithin.com***. This is where you must come to the fork in the road and finally choose how you are going to live your life now.

Will you continue to patty cake with living a healthier life and be comfortable in your uncomfortable state?

Will you tighten up those shoelaces and begin to live a long, fruitful, and joyful life?

I know you can and will make it happen. I love you to life. Let's make it happen!

Your Sister in Christ & Restoration Coach,

Kat

Join the R&R Girlfriends community, receive your "Renew & Restore" Manifesto, and shop at our RFW Marketplace and begin your restoration from within today!

www.RestorationfromWithin.com

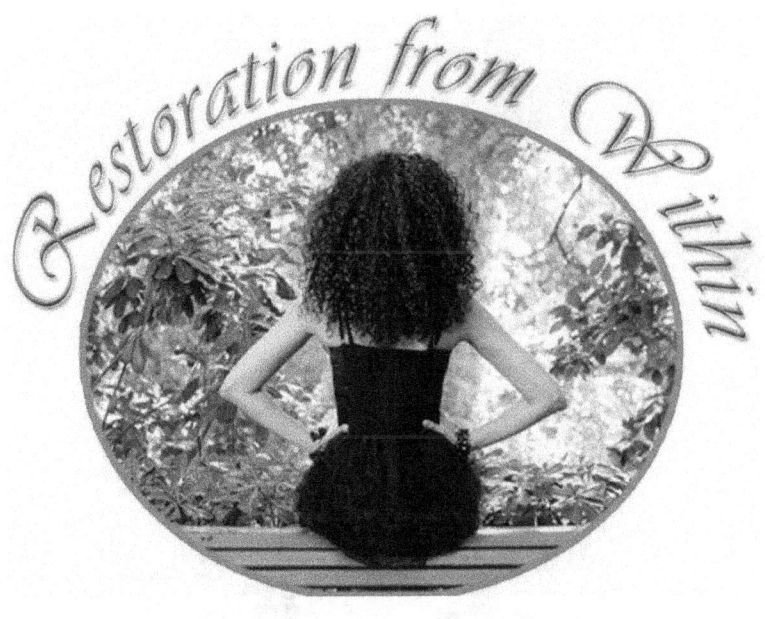

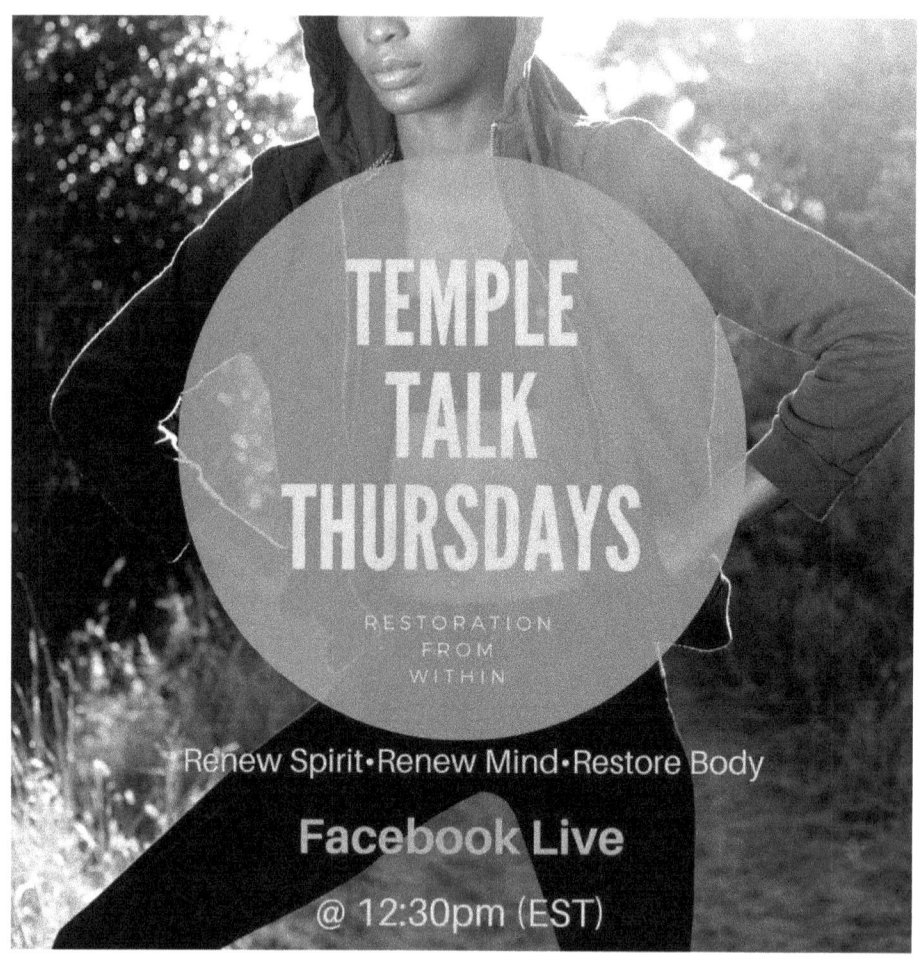

Join us for our Facebook LIVE broadcast **#TempleTalkThursday** at 12:30 pm EST.

Make sure you've "liked" our Restoration from Within page.

Turn on LIVE notifications so that you won't miss the LIVE broadcast.

See you there!

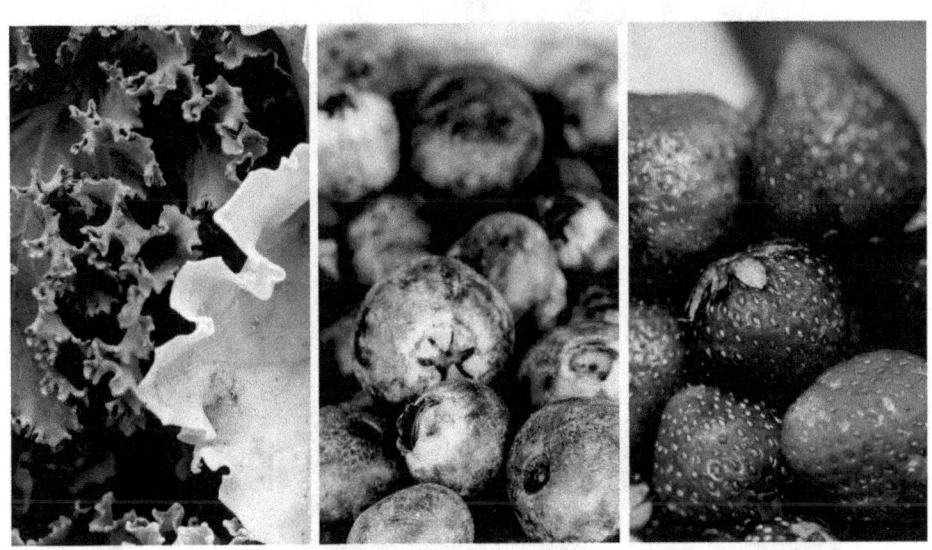

Hit the Refresh Button
GET YOUR RFW JUICE BLENDS TODAY!
WWW.RESTORATIONFROMWITHIN.COM

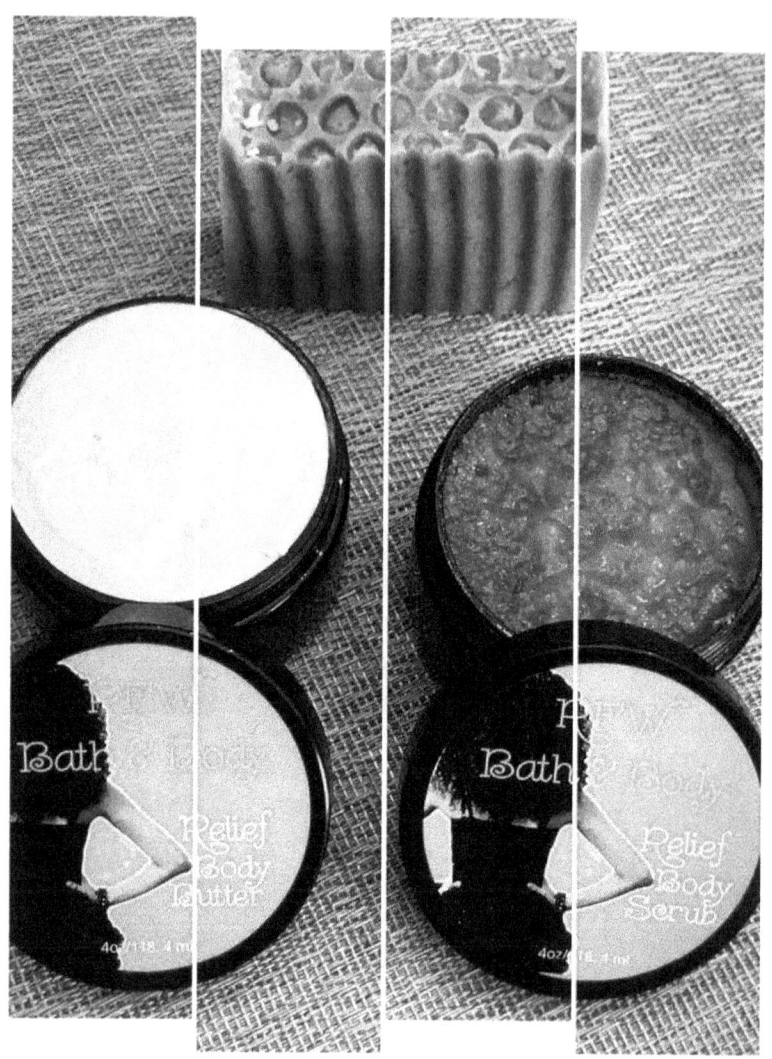

RFW Bath & Body products are handcrafted bath and body products. We select high-quality ingredients so that you can enjoy your cleansing experience with confidence and peace of mind. These products were made to love your body while moisturizing and hydrating your skin. At Restoration from Within we are passionate about restoring and renewing your

Temple from the inside out.

www.ingramcontent.com/pod-product-compliance
Lightning Source LLC
Chambersburg PA
CBHW050655160426
43194CB00010B/1944